D0398023

My (So-Called) Normal Life

My (So-Called) Normal Life

How I learned to balance love, work, family, friends . . . and cancer at 23

ERIN ZAMMETT

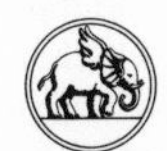

OVERLOOK DUCKWORTH
New York • Woodstock • London

First published in the United States in 2005 by
Overlook Duckworth, Peter Mayer Publishers, Inc.
New York, Woodstock, and London

NEW YORK:
141 Wooster Street
New York, NY 10012

WOODSTOCK:
One Overlook Drive
Woodstock, NY 12498
www.overlookpress.com
[for individual orders, bulk and special sales, contact our Woodstock office]

LONDON:
Duckworth Publishers
90-93 Cowcross Street
London EC1M 6BF
www.ducknet.co.uk
info@duckworth-publishers.co.uk

∞ The paper used in this book meets the requirements for paper permanence as described in the ANSI Z39.48-1992 standard.

Library of Congress Cataloging-in-Publication Data

Zammett, Erin
My (so-called) normal life : how I learned to balance love, work, family, friends—and cancer at 23 / Erin Zammett.
p. cm.
1. Zammett, Erin—Health. 2. Leukemia—Patients—New York (State)—New York—Biography. I. Title: My normal life. II. Title.
RC643.Z36 2005 362.196'99419'0092—dc22 2004066255

Book design and type formatting by Bernard Schleifer
Manufactured in the United States of America
FIRST EDITION
ISBN 1-58567-643-8
ISBN 0-7156-3369-4 (UK)
1 3 5 7 9 8 6 4 2

For my sisters—
Melissa for showing me that when life gives you lemons, you make wine;
and Meghan for always being there to share the bottle.

Contents

My (So-Called) Normal Life

A fork in the road 1

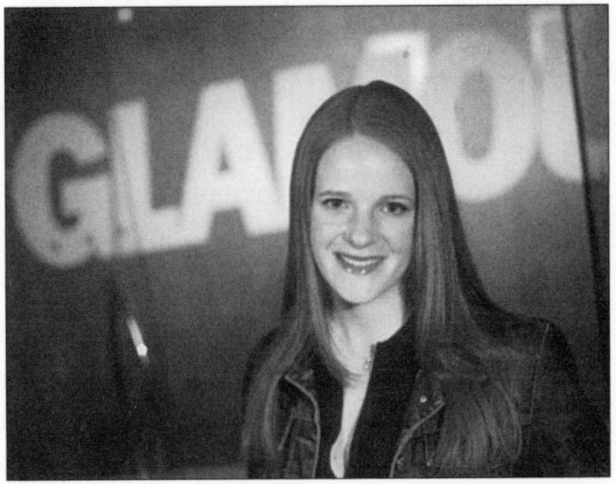

Me, leaving the Glamour offices

I WISH I'D EATEN MORE CHEESEBURGERS. BIG JUICY fat ones with pickles and ketchup and toasted buns. It's not that I like cheeseburgers so much (I'm really more of a chicken girl), it's what they represent to me: joie de vivre, a laid-back, whatever-goes attitude—something I've never had. See, I've always been a control freak, a perfectionist, striving to do and be more every minute of the day. Never quite satisfied. On paper, I had it all: a job at *Glamour* magazine, an awesome boyfriend, a great apartment in New York City, parties to go to almost every night and a supportive, close-knit family nearby. I was living the life I'd always said I wanted. But I was afraid if I slowed down to really enjoy that life, I might not be able to get enough items checked off my to-do list. I might not be a huge success, and nothing could be worse than that. Then, when I was 23, busy plotting my next move, stockpiling my hopes and dreams, I was diagnosed with cancer. So much for my big plans. There is no preparing for news like that, no penciling it in to your otherwise packed schedule. It just happens, without warning. No symptoms, no heads-up, just cancer handed to me on a perfectly nice Tuesday afternoon.

On Monday, November 12, 2001 I went to the doctor for a checkup. I wasn't sick, but I hadn't been to a regular physician in a while so I made an appointment. He was a brand new doctor for me, and I figured it would be a good opportunity to get to know him in case I ever really needed him, for a *real* reason. A friend from work had recommended him: Eric Lutsky, nice, smart, close to the office, took my insurance. Perfect. I also wanted a referral to go to physical therapy for the herniated disc in my back, which I thought was just about the worst thing that could happen to a 23-year-old. I'd been an athlete my whole life—I played Division I volleyball in college—so I'd always taken great care of myself. I ate right, I slept right, I exercised. I figured the doctor would just give me a pat on the back, a "keep up the good work!" Approval and reassurance were two of my favorite things.

The appointment went well. Dr. Lutsky asked me several times if I had any problems, anything bothering me. I felt a little put on the spot, like without a cough or a rash I was wasting this guy's time, but I had nothing to say. I was feeling fine. He explained he would take some blood and run all the standard tests so we could start with a clean slate. Good, I thought. I *was* a little curious about my cholesterol. Not because I worried it was high, but because there was a person in my office who walked around telling everyone how much artery-clogging crap was in every scrap of food they put into their mouths. I wanted so badly to be able to say, "Guess what? I don't care how many LDLs are in this Werther's Original, my cholesterol is, like, two, so back off!"

At the end of the appointment, I said, "So, I'm healthy, right?" He said, "Yup." Check that off my list. I told him it was nice to meet him, he said likewise and I left. The nurse gave me a card and told me I could call the following Monday for my lab work. I marked it in my calendar, walked outside with my clean bill of health and grabbed a cab back to work.

For the next 24 hours, I went about my life as usual: work, gym, frozen burrito, *Road Rules*. Then I got the call that would change everything. I had just returned from lunch with a book publicist (I was technically an editorial assistant at *Glamour*, the lowest on the totem pole, but I was editing our books coverage, so I got wined and dined a lot) and there was a message on my voicemail from Dr. Lutsky. As soon as I heard his voice, I held my breath—why was he calling me? For a second I thought he might be reminding me to fax the results of my MRI so he could write the referral for physical therapy. But then I realized doctors never call patients themselves for silly administrative things. Shit, what could this be?

The message went on: He got my labs back and had a question, could I give him a call back? My heart plunged and my mind scrolled through a list of worst-case scenarios as I started dialing. Could it be my cholesterol? Would he call for that or have his nurse call? Maybe it's really, really high. I could go on a no-fat diet. Sure I would miss chips and salsa, but it's not the end of the world. And I'd finally be able to lose the five pounds that I didn't really need to lose. I dialed his number and waited. I know! Oh my God I must be pregnant! Holy shit. I traced the past month—had I missed a pill? What would I do, I'm only 23! My life was going so well. But what if it's something worse? Something way worse and God would punish me for thinking that a baby would be the end of my life. What if it's so bad that I *wished* I were just pregnant?

Dr. Lutsky was with a patient and he'd have to call me back. Great, more time to what-if. I wrote a thank-you email to the publicist for the lunch, and pretended not to worry, but I couldn't even feel my fingers punching the keys. I just knew something was wrong, and I wondered if my coworkers could tell. I sat in a part of the office called "the pod," an open, newsroom-style area right outside of the editor-in-chief's office. There were no walls, no doors and no more than two feet between editors. It was by far the coolest, most tuned-in place to sit, but it was a bit of a three-ring circus at times. Donald, the magazine's creative director, who despite being the number two person at *Glamour*, chose to sit in the pod, was constantly shouting a request for something—a reservation at Odeon, a "girl" dollar bill (crisp enough for the vending machine to accept it), the spelling of the word "tomorrow." And there was always, *always* food lying around—ice cream cake for someone's birthday, a pizza that the fashion department couldn't possibly finish, a tray of bagels and fruit from a meeting that got cancelled. Editors from other areas of the office came by to graze—and to check out the pod's giveaway tables that overflowed with books, CDs, lipsticks and, occasionally, half-eaten sandwiches that Julie, our photo researcher, didn't have the heart to throw away. The pod was fun—and sometimes productive—but it was not the ideal place to have a serious chat with your doctor.

Finally, my phone rang. I told Dr. Lutsky I'd call him right back from a private office. I ran in and dialed with a shaky hand. He got on the line (after his assistant tried to tell me he was with a patient again!) and in a calm and soothing voice asked how I was doing. "I feel like I'm going to puke," I said. He said he understood, and then told me why he was calling: My white blood cell count was very high (a normal person's is between 4,000 and 10,000; mine was well over 70,000). This would usually signal an infection, but I was perfectly healthy. And my LDH levels were abnormal too. I had no idea what an LDH was so Dr. Lutsky translated: "It's not good," he said, "but I don't want to make a statement until we take more blood and run the tests again to be sure it's not a mistake." Not good? Make a statement? It all sounded so doctorly and serious. Then he said,

"Erin, I don't think this should wait. Can you come down right away?"

With my jacket still on, I went to my boss, Alison, and said casually, "Hi there, I'm back from lunch but I have to go to the doctor now. I got some abnormal blood tests back." The second part of that statement was choked out through tears. She handed me a tissue and asked questions I didn't have the answers to. It could be anything, we agreed, but we both knew that when your doctor *tells* you it isn't good, it probably isn't good. Then we both cried. Over the past year, we had gotten very close. Sure, I answered her phones and opened her mail—and even got her salami and cheese paninis sometimes—but we also confided in each other. We talked about our love lives and our families and friends almost as much as we talked about work. She told me to take the afternoon off, which freaked me out—what was this guy going to tell me that would require me to take the afternoon off? I went back to my desk and called my mom to let her know what was going on. She was her normal distracted work self, talking to three people at once, listening to me with half an ear. But she didn't seem worried, which made me less so. (She later told me that the minute she heard abnormal blood, she knew it was bad.) We hung up and I hurried out the door.

Back in Dr. Lutsky's waiting room, I tried to keep my mind occupied. I sat there long enough to read through half of an old issue of *Shape* magazine. I remember thinking that the people in their weight loss story weren't that impressive, that their "after" pictures didn't look so different from their "before" shots and that we would never have put them in *Glamour*. Then I felt bad and thought maybe I shouldn't be so shallow at a time like this. The women looked nice. They looked happy and healthy. I thought good thoughts, and hoped that would somehow affect my prognosis, like a last-minute kiss-up to God or whoever it is that hands out terminal illnesses.

It didn't work. Dr. Lutsky took me into an exam room and

sat me on the table. He checked my spleen and my lymph nodes and shrugged; they seemed fine to him. Had I been tired? he asked. Lost a lot of weight lately? Ha! I wish. What about night sweats? Fever? No, I said. What I felt like saying is, "Um, hello, I was here yesterday, I was the one in perfect health, remember???" Instead I asked him what he thought was wrong with me, but he didn't want to get into it. The nurse took more blood and we made an appointment for Thursday morning; it would take 36 hours to get the results back. He said he thought my parents should come too, if I was OK with that. My parents had to be there? Oh my God, this *was* serious. I couldn't leave without knowing what he was going to tell us, so I kept asking questions, hoping he'd get a little more specific. Eventually I wore him down. He said he thought it was an infection in the blood. I immediately thought HIV (never mind that I hadn't been given an AIDS test). I would kill my boyfriend, Nick. But he'd been tested. Or did he lie? Oh my God, what if I have AIDS?

We kept talking. I told the doctor I'd had a blood disorder once before—idiopathic thrombocytopenic purpura (ITP). It's a rare autoimmune-related disease that I had when I was eight. I spent two weeks in the hospital getting steroids pumped into me, then went right back to the third grade where my class threw me a cupcake party. I never had a problem again.

"Could it be that?" I asked.

"This isn't ITP," he said, with a look that read, "you *wish* this was ITP, honey."

"Well what are we talking about then?" I pressed.

"We're talking about a blood infection," he said.

He was being so vague I wanted to scream, but I could tell he was ready to put an end to our silly little game, so I continued.

"Like what kind of blood infection?"

Silence.

"Like *leukemia*?" I asked, with the slightly embarrassed

uncertainty I felt in school when I thought I knew the answer, but just wasn't sure.

"Yes," he said, "like leukemia."

Aha! I got it out of him! I win! But now I wanted to put it back. I just nodded my head and said, "Wow." If I tried to say anything more, I knew sobs would come out instead of words, and I couldn't bear to break down in front of a guy I barely knew. It was probably hard enough for him already, having to tell a patient she had cancer 24 hours after meeting her—(and telling her she was perfectly healthy). Dr. Lutsky still didn't want to "say" anything until we got the new results back, just in case it was a mistake. But he quickly added that he didn't think it was. Then he said, "Coming to my office yesterday may have been the best thing you've ever done for yourself." It sounded like a line from the *Lifetime* movie of the week or a *Dateline* special. It was all too weird, too familiar. I cried, and then laughed at myself for crying. He gave me a tissue and told me to try to relax. And not to drink any alcohol. He'd see me Thursday morning. This was bad, very bad.

I can handle this, I thought, as I walked out of his office. I had no idea what it was I'd have to handle but I told myself I could do it. In a way, I was prepared for something like this, expecting it even. My whole life I'd lain awake at night having horrible thoughts about my parents and my grandparents and my sisters—plane crashes, car crashes, heart attacks, cancer. My family had it pretty good, and I always felt like our number would have to be up sooner or later, like it was only a matter of time before the dreaded phone call came. I just never thought I'd be the one that call was about.

Desperate to talk to my mom, I scanned the streets for a payphone. Of course I had walked out of my apartment without my cell phone that morning. I crossed the street and fumbled through my bag for some change.

"He thinks it could be something bad," I told her, unable to just say the word.

"Did he say what?" she asked.

"Yes," I said.

"What did he *say*, Erin?" she was getting annoyed.

"He said that it wasn't good, and it could be really bad if it wasn't a mistake," I said, desperately trying to come up with a way to sugarcoat the news. I suddenly understood how Dr. Lutsky must have felt.

"How bad, Erin?" she pressed.

I leaned into the phone booth and whispered, not wanting anyone—especially myself—to hear me say the words out loud.

"Like . . . leukemia, Mom."

And just like that, it was real. "What?" my mom shrieked. "Holy shit. What's the doctor's number?" She sounded like she was going to yell at him, like it was his fault. Then we were interrupted: "Please deposit 10 cents. Ten cents please." I pumped dimes into the phone and tried to relay every detail. On the third interruption by the operator, my mom got really frustrated. "Don't you have a goddamn quarter?" she fumed. I knew she wasn't mad, just scared, like the time she yelled at me for getting lost on our Brownie field trip to Radio City Music Hall (I hadn't actually been lost, I just followed the other leader into the bathroom without telling my mom). I told her that Dr. Lutsky didn't want to talk until he knew more, and that I wished she wouldn't bother him. But I knew she'd call. She'd ask a million questions and get some answers too. Then she'd talk to more doctors. My mom works in a hospital and makes friends with every janitor, X-ray technician and surgeon she meets. She was going to use her connections.

My mom is a tough lady, and she's great in emergencies—medical, fashion and otherwise. She always knows the right thing to do or say and manages to stay relatively calm. In a crisis, my two sisters and I would usually go to my mom, who's the far more rational of our two parents. Then she'd decide if it was worth telling my dad. Certain things—my 12 parking tickets sophomore year, Meghan's shamrock tattoo, the price of Melissa's wedding dress—were better kept between the girls. My dad is a complete alarmist and just a tad temperamental. When Meghan, my younger sister, tore up her knee on a ski slope in Vermont a few years back, my dad was so upset, he took her skis, snapped them in half over his knee and heaved them into the woods. He hasn't skied since. My mom and I decided it would be best if we waited until my dad was back from his business trip to tell him in person. We hung up and I headed back to work.

As people on the sidewalk bumped past me with cigarettes burning, I wanted to shout, watch where you put that thing, I have cancer! But I had a sudden sympathy for these strangers. Who knew what was going on in their lives, if they had just gotten similar news. I certainly looked like a normal person, but I wasn't. Not anymore. I put on my sunglasses and let myself cry.

When I got back to the office, I checked my face in the bathroom mirror (I remember thinking how green my eyes looked from all the tears) and went right into Alison's office. It had only been an hour since I told her about my bad blood and now I had answers. "He's pretty sure I have leukemia," I said, my voice cracking. We both cried, and laughed a bit imagining Donald drawing one of his famous caricatures for me. He'd make me tall and thin (as all of his females were—no wonder we all loved him) with no hair. Cancer Girl, he'd call it. "You should go home," Alison said. "And don't worry about coming in tomorrow." But it was only Tuesday and I didn't have my appointment with Dr. Lutsky until Thursday. What else would I do? I told Alison I'd see her in the morning and went back to my desk to close up for the day. I really wanted to talk to my boyfriend Nick, but my mom had convinced me to wait to tell him later that night, in person. Back then, he was not my first call when things went wrong—or right, for that matter. My parents were. My sisters and I talked to them often and about everything. Sure they offered their opinion even when it wasn't asked for, but for the most part they just wanted to help. And we let them. Though my dependence on my parents usually pissed Nick off, I knew he'd appreciate it in this case.

Nick and I had been together a little over two years when I was diagnosed. I met him in the beginning of my senior year at The University of Tennessee. He'd just moved to Knoxville from Michigan to live with friends after an unsuccessful freshman stint at Central Michigan University (the details of which I didn't learn about until some time later). Nick was tall, dark, handsome and from the North, which, after spending three years chasing thick-accented Southern boys in frayed baseball hats, was like a godsend to me. Our backgrounds were completely different; he grew up in a low-income neighborhood in Flint, Michigan, where he got jumped by high school gangs; I grew up in an upper-middle class neighborhood on Long Island where we didn't lock our doors at night. But we complemented each other perfectly. He got me to plan less and live more, sleep past 7:30 on the weekends, skip the gym every once in a while. I encouraged him to use his potential, to play a little less Frisbee golf, smoke a little less pot (I'd always been attracted to charming underachievers). When we were together, we were the best versions of ourselves.

Nick was close to his family, but he didn't count on them for financial support, so he'd been working various jobs since he was 14, which made him seem more grown up and more independent than most guys I knew. Though he was often too cool for school—literally—he was a complete goofball when he was around me. Even when we were doing nothing, we had a great time. And we wanted the same things from life—to be smart, to be successful professionally and to be surrounded by family and friends (and to have enough money to go on great vacations and eat at nice restaurants). After I graduated and moved to New

York City, we spent a year doing the long-distance thing. Then he moved up to New York too. He signed up for classes at a local college, took a job with my father's company and crashed at my parents' house until he could find a place of his own. For some people, having your boyfriend live with your parents would be out of the question, way too close for comfort. In my family, it wasn't weird at all.

My parents live in Huntington, a beautiful town on the north shore of Long Island, about an hour outside of the city. They've been in the same house for over 30 years and though my sisters and I didn't technically live there anymore, we still hung around all the time. As did half the neighborhood. On any given night there was action at the Zammett house—a neighbor stops by to return a ladder and stays for a glass of wine; a cousin drops off a freshly-caught fish and stays to fry it up (and drink a glass of wine); My older sister, Melissa, and her fiance show up for steak (and wine) and wind up sleeping over. There was always a party going on, but there was also always work to be done. Whether it was the basement flooding again and needing to be pumped, or the pool needing to be uncovered, or covered, or cleaned, or the 300 beer bottles from a backyard party needing to be recycled, there was some project being done that required manpower. And my parents had no problem asking anyone who happened to be there to help. When our friends came over in high school they knew they ran the risk of being put to work, but they also knew they'd eat good food and have a great time. "Never a dull moment" as my mother likes to say. With the constant flow of craziness, Nick simply blended in.

I looked at the work scattered across my desk—half-written articles, a pile of messages to be returned, dog-eared book catalogs—and it all seemed so foreign. Like it belonged to a different girl, a girl who three hours earlier had a different life. I wondered if any of it mattered anymore, if I'd even be coming back. I got the job at *Glamour* a few months after I graduated, and I'd been there a little over a year and a half when I was diagnosed. I'd wanted to be a writer ever since my short story "Mrs. Peach and the Magic Cereal Box" won first place in the second-grade writing contest, and I loved magazines so it seemed like the perfect career. Of course I wasn't writing award-winning features—and no job is as glamorous as it sounds—but I was happy there. And I had it pretty good. Late nights, but fancy lunches; a tiny paycheck, but free lip gloss. But now I had cancer. I tied up a few loose ends and told Jaimee, my pod mate and friend, what was going on. We sat close enough to each other to hear what the other was thinking, but we mostly communicated through email (a necessity with all the eager ears in the pod). She had sent me one saying, "Are you OK?" I had to tell her no. First she was outraged on my behalf: "Who the hell is this doctor? Are you getting a second opinion?" Then she said it would be OK. Her uncle had leukemia so she knew a lot about it.

"How is he doing?" I asked.

"Um, he died," she said.

I would find this scenario repeating itself again and again as I told more people about my diagnosis. I think it's just human nature for people to try to relate, to respond to my cancer news by telling me about someone *they* know with the disease. Occasionally, though, they'd forget to filter out the anecdotes about people who didn't fare so well. It was harmless, really. More upsetting for them because they'd think they just told me something I didn't already know: that I might die, too.

I decided to go my parents' house for the night. Nick would be there, of course, and Melissa and her fiance, Ysrael, lived right around the corner. I could tell them all in person in one fell swoop. They could see for themselves that I was perfectly fine, that I was going to be fine. At the train station, I bought a $6 *Martha Stewart* Christmas cookie magazine and accidentally left it at the kiosk. Does life get any crueler? Cancer

I could handle; having nothing to read on an hour-long train ride after being diagnosed with that cancer was torture. I called Lucy, one of my oldest and best friends. Her dad had died in the World Trade Center on September 11th so things had been pretty awful for her the past two months. I hadn't planned to tell anyone until I had more details, but in some ways I felt like my news would take her mind off her dad, if only for a few minutes. It would give her something else to focus on, someone *she* could feel sorry for, since I knew she was tired of being the object of everyone's sympathy. Plus I was dying to tell someone. We talked for a minute and I told her I'd call as soon as I knew anything, then we went into the tunnel under the East River and my phone cut out.

After spending the better half of the ride picturing myself bald—would I wear scarves? A wig? Would I leave the house?—I decided to call Melissa. I just couldn't help myself. In some ways keeping quiet about my potential diagnosis was like having really good gossip and not spilling it. I *wanted* to tell people. She was on her cell phone on her way home from work. I cupped my hand over the receiver and said, "I think I have leukemia." She couldn't hear me so I had to repeat myself about seven times. Then she went into a dead zone and I lost her.

My mom picked me up from the train station and we stopped at Tortilla Grill to get some healthy burritos for dinner (I got loaded nachos on the side—since it was likely I had cancer, I figured I could live a little). Being able to pick out the dinner for the family made me feel oddly special, and a little sad. Growing up we had a home-cooked, sit-down meal every single night, but we certainly didn't have a say in what that meal was. If beef stroganoff and lima beans were on the menu, we ate beef stroganoff and lima beans. Except when it was your birthday. Or if you broke a bone. Then my mom would make you whatever you wanted. On birthdays, I chose chicken francese and spaghetti, which was so buttery I'd leave the table with a shiny chin. When I broke my arm playing soccer in the 4th grade and my collarbone playing bike tag in 8th, I opted for chicken tenders and fries with honey from Burger King. And Coke. My sisters and I didn't get junk food on a regular basis, so whenever the opportunity presented itself, we jumped all over it. But now that I was an adult and it wasn't my birthday and I didn't just break my leg, I wanted someone to argue with me, to say *not* Mexican, *Chinese*. But no one did, because no one wanted to upset me. So far only my mom and Melissa knew, but they were both being alarmingly nice. We're a bunch of fiery redheads. Normally, we're competitive, we argue, we fight. Sure we love each other—probably more than any family I've ever known—but "nice" is just not a word I'd use to describe the way we interact with one another.

As it turned out, there was a particularly affectionate houseguest staying at my parents' that night—typical—and I didn't feel like getting any more hugs, so we headed to Melissa and Ysrael's apartment. Nick was at class. I called him on his cell phone and told him I was in Huntington for the night, which made him happy. I worked long hours at *Glamour* and he was working full time and taking a full course load, so we didn't see much of each other during the week. Then I told him why I was there. "They think it's leukemia," I said. We didn't talk long. He was at Melissa's apartment 40 minutes later (he said he drove 100 miles an hour, which I don't doubt). My stomach dropped when I heard him walking up the stairs. I was nervous to see him. I hated being sappy and sentimental, but when you've just found out that you have some crazy disease and you don't know what happens next, there's really no avoiding it. I got up, met him at the door and we just hugged. His whole body started shaking, and I realized he was crying, sobbing. He held me so tight. I cried too.

Then we walked back into the living room, dug into our dinner and had a fairly normal night. We're not a "let's talk about our feelings" kind of family—I'd rarely seen my mother cry (something that changed very quickly after I was diagnosed), and I'd *never* seen my father cry—and we certainly didn't feel bad for ourselves. But cancer was new territory for us. Could we just buck up and handle it like we'd handle any other obstacle? With hard work, humor and a lot of wine? Are you allowed to drink when you have cancer? Are you allowed to laugh about cancer? Did life go on? We were all clueless.

Melissa was getting married soon and was very concerned about my being able to be in her wedding—a day she'd been planning since she was 5. She had just met Ysrael a year earlier while vacationing with her best friend, Sherry, in Venezuela—he was the "director of fun," or something like that, at the all-inclusive hotel where they were staying. Melissa fell madly in love at first sight, as she had been known to do, and called us all to share the good news. His name was Drop Dead Gorgeous, or at least that's what she was calling him. We all wrote it off as another one of her unrequited crushes (he hadn't given her the time of day yet) until a month later when she booked another trip to Venezuela to visit him. Then a few months after that—after racking up thousands of dollars in international phone calls—she was back in Venezuela again. That time Ysrael proposed on the beach at sunset. My parents were there too. They had gone down to meet him and so that he could ask for my father's permission—it was all pretty well-orchestrated by Melissa. She is the polar opposite of me. She knows what she wants, she goes after it and she never second-guesses herself. To her, everything is black and white (no wonder she became an accountant). But she's also completely able to go with the flow, she loves to party and is almost always happy. I hate her for that sometimes. Anyway, after months of jumping through the government's red tape, Ysrael, who's Catholic, not Jewish—his mother had him when she was 17; her family was fighting so she named him Ysrael because there were wars going on in Israel at the time, or so the story goes—was finally in the U.S. and the wedding was set. All of our heads were still spinning. Did she really know this guy? He barely spoke English. What would he do for work? But nothing, not even my leukemia-ridden body, was going to ruin her big day. She joked that she'd wheel me down the aisle if she had to. Melissa was a bit of a bridezilla—when one of her bridesmaids didn't fit into her dress, Melissa promptly left work in the middle of the day, picked up her friend and drove straight to Weight Watchers—so I knew she was serious.

But the truth was, none of us had any idea what was going to happen to me. I could be in the hospital by then, or worse. But we didn't talk about that. We just popped in a movie—*America's Sweethearts*—and laughed a lot, as we tended to do when things sucked. After the movie, which also sucked, we went home and went to bed. I was allowed to sleep with Nick, who incidentally, was living in my old bedroom, surrounded by my volleyball trophies and prom pictures and stuffed animals my high school boyfriend had given me. (OK, so maybe the situation was a little weird.) Normally, we had to stay in separate bedrooms but, again, no one wanted to upset the cancer patient. If I'd asked my mom for $10,000 that night she would've gotten out her checkbook.

"I'm really scared," I confided to Nick before we fell asleep.

"I know," he said. "Me too."

Then he told me that everything was going to be OK, that *I* was going to be OK. But I wasn't sure either of us believed it. He wrapped me in his arms and we laid there silently, tears streaming down our faces. I slept like a baby that night, so calm it was frightening. But I suppose it made sense. I was someone who totally sweated all the small stuff, but suddenly there was no small stuff to lose sleep over. There was just one big thing: cancer. And that was out of my control.

The next morning, I had tears in my eyes before I even opened them. But I knew it wasn't all just a nightmare. In fact I already couldn't remember what it was like to not have cancer. From the second the word leukemia came out of Dr. Lutsky's mouth, that's all I knew. I got on the treadmill and walked very slowly—I suddenly felt fragile, like the tiniest jolt could upset the rogue cells swimming in my bloodstream. I wanted to be a good patient, but I had no idea what that meant. At the train station, I grabbed a bagel and a container of orange juice (which I don't like, but seemed like a healthy idea) and headed back under the East River, back into the city, back to work. When I got there I returned a few emails and tried to avoid my coworkers—other than Alison and Jaimee, none of them knew yet, which was bizarre. It was like I had wandered on to a movie set but no one noticed I didn't belong so they just acted around me.

My phone rang and my dad's cell number popped up on the caller ID. He was still in Vegas for his business trip and had no idea what was going on. I almost didn't pick up, but then my morbid imagination kicked in—what if he gets in a plane crash and this was my last opportunity to talk to him and I missed it? I conjured up a cheery voice and said hello. He had just boarded his plane home and was calling to see how I was doing and to tell me about some super fast car he got to drive. He owns a small computer sales company and was in Vegas for a big convention. One of his clients took him to the Shelby car factory where they took a ride in a Cobra and he thought that was the neatest thing in the world.

My dad and I were really tight; we'd stay at the dinner table long after the dishes had been cleared just talking and dreaming about the future. Neither of us could sit still in life, so we related that way. He pushed me to be better, smarter. He had been everywhere and done everything and tried to pass on what he'd learned to my sisters and me. Every night he'd tuck us in and we'd play guessing games—picture Trivial Pursuit for a four, eight and ten-year-old. He'd ask us random questions about geography, anatomy, sports or our own lives: "Who can tell me the name of the boat where we had brunch in Disney World last year?" he'd ask as if he were a real game show host. I lived for that time of day. Usually, Melissa and I, who are only two years apart, competed, and Meghan, who is four years younger than me, got some throwaway question like, "What color is the sky?" Sometimes, if we couldn't come up with the answer, he'd leave us to think about it overnight. I'd fall asleep racking my little brain, desperately trying to come up with the answer to both beat my big sister and impress my dad. He's a tough guy to please, so when you got his approval, when you made him proud, you knew you were special. The boat, by the way, was called the Empress Lily.

When he asked me how I was doing, I felt so guilty not telling him what was going on.

I felt worse knowing that he would never be this happy again, that once he landed in New York, he'd learn that his invincible daughter was sick. In some ways I felt like I had let him down. I was the one with all the plans, the one who was going to make it big. It never occurred to either of us that I couldn't do or be anything I wanted. But now that hardly seemed possible.

Our weekly magazine status meeting—where we all get called out for missing deadlines—is torturous even when you're not waiting around for your doctor to tell you that you do indeed have cancer. Unable to feign interest in where the layout was for the "Three Life-Threatening Diseases Your Doctor May Not Be Telling You About" feature, I let myself zone out. I tried to imagine what a life with cancer would be like. I pictured myself bald and skinny with grayish-green skin. A high school friend of mine had recently had leukemia and was bald, skinny and gray, so I had a working knowledge of the ickiness I could expect. But he'd done exceptionally well and was in remission. My first cancer role model. I traced back the past few weeks to figure out when, exactly, I came down with this thing. Did I have it when I was shopping on Fifth Avenue that day with Amy? My legs *were* really tired. What about last week when Tim and I got drunk on vodka tonics at that book party? Did the alcohol make it worse? I wondered if I'd have to leave New York City, give everything up, move back in with my parents.

After the meeting, I called my mom just to check in. She had been trying all morning to get back the results of my blood test—she wasn't going to wait until Thursday for an answer so she found an oncologist who was willing to read the lab report right away. She was crying.

"It's not good," she said. She had just spoken to Dr. Lutsky, who'd already conferred with the oncologist.

"You have chronic myelogenous leukemia," she said.

I started crying.

"Is that bad?" I asked.

All she'd gleaned from the conversation with the oncologist was that it's a type of leukemia that most commonly affects older people, the only known cure is a bone marrow transplant and there's some new drug called Gleevec that I might be able to take. Oh, and no more appointment with Dr. Lutsky. I needed to have a bone marrow biopsy to confirm the diagnosis and to find out what phase I was in. It was on to the big dogs now.

The name Gleevec sounded oddly familiar. When I went to Alison's office to update her, she couldn't believe the eerie coincidence. *Glamour* had just done a story on chronic myelogenous leukemia and Gleevec in the December 2001 issue, which had just hit newsstands that day. It was called "These Women Knew They Were Dying . . . Then a New Drug Saved Their Lives." Not exactly beach reading, I thought. I hadn't read the story yet, and had I not been diagnosed, I probably wouldn't have. I wasn't very good with disease and death.

Hospitals depressed me—I couldn't even watch commercials for *ER*—and if the topic of death came up, I changed the subject. But now I couldn't avoid it. I took a copy of the issue to read later and went to tell our editor-in-chief, Cindi Leive, about my diagnosis. The *Glamour* grapevine, which was really just one over-excited editor, had already reached her so she knew, but she still looked floored. She told me not to worry about any of my work and that I could use her private bathroom and the VIP car service whenever I needed it. Would I need to use her bathroom? Yikes. She was incredibly nice and down-to-earth and completely approachable, but I couldn't imagine walking into the editor-in-chief's office to throw up (or whatever it was I'd be doing in my new role as cancer patient). She hugged me and I started to cry. And then I laughed. I'd never been a big crier and suddenly I was weeping uncontrollably every five minutes.

Work may not seem like the ideal place to be when you find out you have cancer, but for me it was a blessing. The editor who worked on the Gleevec story gave me all sorts of information, including the name and number of the man who developed the drug. Cindi helped me get an appointment at Memorial Sloan-Kettering Cancer Center, which is *the* place to be if you've got cancer, and Jaimee bought me two bags of Pirate's Booty for the train ride back to Huntington. I was ready.

That night my dad arrived home from his business trip. My mom met him at the airport, crying before he even got through the gates. He handled it well, she told me later, and I didn't press her for details. The only one left to tell was Meghan, who was at The University of Tennessee studying for finals. She'd decided to go to Tennessee after visiting me there a few times—all of which were spent drinking and kissing much older guys. When she first started there, I drove her to the mall, brought her to the best off-campus parties and got her into the coolest bars. What I should have done was help her with her homework. The weekend I graduated, with aunts and uncles and cousins in town, we found out that Meghan had gotten a 1.7 for her first year at UT. Not exactly acceptable. So in between my commencement ceremony and my party, my dad raced like a madman—temper flaring—to pick up a U-Haul. He spent much of the rest of the weekend "packing her little ass up." She was moving home. Grades were very important in my family, and Meghan needed to learn that. Being the youngest, she definitely had it the easiest, but in some ways she was cheated because she wasn't pushed (case in point: What color is the sky?). She was also allowed to quit—soccer, Girl Scouts, ballet—which for Melissa and me, was never an option. Meghan was fragile, she didn't like to sweat, she had pet mice. At the dinner table, Melissa and I tag-teamed the conversation, talking about her latest crush or our most awful teachers ever or the big game I had coming up. If Meghan opened her mouth, she was usually interrupted or just talked over by Melissa or me, who thought what we had to say was more important (and in our defense, it usually was). My mom hated that we didn't give Meghan a chance and always tried to run interference. To this day, if Meghan opens her mouth at the dinner table, even if it's just to ask someone to pass the salt, my mom says, "Everyone shush, Meghan has something to say."

After doing a semester at a community college on Long Island and pulling her grades up, she was back at Tennessee, in her second year. She was doing better, but it was still touch and go. Finding out her big sister had cancer wouldn't likely help her concentration, so we agreed it would be best to wait until the weekend to break the news to her.

The appointment at Sloan-Kettering was set for the next morning. My first official cancer meeting and I still felt perfectly healthy! I kept waiting for my body to catch up and shut down, to start acting like it had cancer. But it didn't. It was all happening so fast. One minute I was stressing about getting a full workout in before meeting my friends for drinks; now I was worrying about getting a second opinion on my life. I wanted so badly to go back to before I was diagnosed and cut myself some slack, enjoy the life I had because I knew it would never be the same. But it was too late.

Cancer 101 2

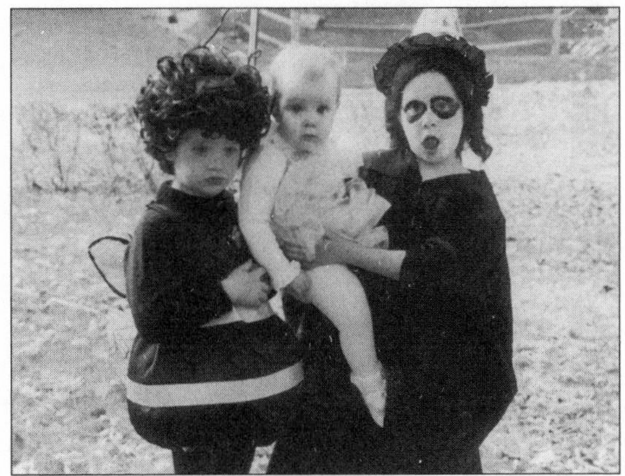

My sisters and me (the bee) on Halloween

JUST WALKING THROUGH THE DOORS AT MEMORIAL Sloan-Kettering made me feel better. Doctors and nurses were bustling around, clipboards in hand; receptionists were calling out patients' names; pharmacists were churning out prescriptions at a rapid pace. It looked like the kind of place where things get done, and it didn't have that antiseptic hospital smell, which was a huge plus. Don't get me wrong, there were plenty of people wheeling around with tubes sticking out of their necks and arms, wearing scarves and baseball caps to cover their bald heads. But still, I was glad we were there, relieved to be with people who knew what they were talking about, people who had the answers to my questions. Sure I appreciated Melissa and Nick telling me I was going to be OK, that I'd beat this thing, but I wanted to hear it from someone in a white coat.

My parents, Nick and I got a crash course in chronic myelogenous leukemia, CML, from Kathleen Cathcart, my new oncologist. It had only been 48 hours since I was at little old Dr. Lutsky's office on 36th and Madison and now I had my very own oncologist. Very strange, and a little depressing. When we got into the car that morning to head to the train station, there'd been a commercial for a cancer institute blaring on the radio. How appropriate, I thought. But no one said anything. And no one lowered the volume. We just sat there for a second, one big not-so happy family in uncomfortable silence.

It hadn't occurred to me that Nick would come to the appointment, but he said he wanted to and was insulted when I acted surprised by that. I just didn't think he needed to be there. He was my best friend—and we knew everything about each other—but having an entourage made me feel worse, like I wasn't capable of hearing what the doctor had to say on my own, like there was something really wrong with me. Having my dad there was going to be hard enough. It wasn't that I thought he'd try to snap the doctor's stethoscope in two or kick in the exam table; I just didn't want to see him sad. I knew he already felt like he had failed in some way, like he couldn't protect me from this.

My father's father died when my dad was in his twenties. Since then he'd been watching out for his mother and three sisters. Add a wife and three daughters, throw in a business to run and he was under a lot of pressure. He's a control freak just like me (or rather, I'm just like him) so he can be a total asshole sometimes, suck the wind right out of your sails. But he just likes to be in charge, to help people. And he's good at it. Before he got into the computer business, my father had been an air-traffic controller and he treats life with the same intensity. If the neighbor's son needs to borrow golf clubs, my dad will come home from his office and personally fit him with one of the five sets he keeps in the basement. If you need directions somewhere, my dad is the guy to call. He could give you 17 ways to get from point A to point B without hitting a single red light—or a pothole. People call him for job advice, restaurant recommendations, fishing tips. But cancer was a different story. He didn't have the answer, and I knew that would crush him. If there had been a way to keep the whole thing from him, I would have done it.

There was a little food cart in the hospital lobby where we got Starbucks coffee, bananas and gourmet muffins before heading to the leukemia floor (I couldn't decide if having a whole floor dedicated to people like me was reassuring or terrifying). My mom was able to use her Huntington Hospital ID card, so she got everything for like $2, which she thought was very cool, perhaps a sign that things might not be so bad after all. She loves a deal.

Up on the fourth floor, I got my finger pricked and filled out some paperwork. Then we all filed into the exam room and the nurse checked my vital signs (still alive!) and weighed me—this seemed unnecessary and a little cruel, but I didn't say anything. I wanted to be a model patient. I wanted these people to like me. The nurse asked me some questions about my life. Do I smoke? Do I have sex? Do I live on a nuclear power plant? Standard, really. Then Dr. Cathcart came in and we all sat at attention like eager students on the first day of school. Today's lesson: cancer at 23.

Dr. Cathcart was young, pretty and female, which somehow made me feel better, like maybe we'd be on the same side, friends even. It always surprised me when super-smart, super-specialized doctors looked like people you might bump into on the sidewalk, or work out next to at the gym, like when you discovered one of your elementary school teachers' first names, or saw them at the grocery store. (Wait a minute, Isn't your first name Mr.? Don't you live at the school? Mommy!) She didn't schmooze us at all, which was good for my dad since he was there for the facts. I wouldn't have minded a "so how was the ride in?" or "what's the weather like out there?" Something to take the edge off. But this wasn't the time for small talk.

Here's what we got instead: CML is a chronic form of leukemia, meaning it moves slowly. And it appeared that mine was in the early phase—it wasn't going to kill me the next day or even the day after that. I can handle slow-moving, I thought. So far, so good. But, she added, I'd probably had the disease for some time now without knowing it (most CML patients don't know they have the disease until they go to the doctor for something else—thank God Dr. Lutsky had been so thorough). My white blood cell count had jumped from 70,000 to 98,000 in the past two days, so it was only a matter of time before the symptoms kicked in. This completely freaked me out. I must have had it last month at Amanda's bachelorette party, I thought. But I'd had so much fun. It didn't make any sense. Then she continued: CML cannot be stopped with traditional chemotherapy and radiation. And the only known cure is a bone marrow transplant, a grueling procedure that requires a genetically-matched donor and has about a 15 percent mortality rate (and completely zaps your fertility). Historically, CML is treated with the drugs Interferon and Ara-C, both given in injection form, both involving horrible side effects like depression, flu-like illness and crippling fatigue. And those only work in about 30 percent of patients. Left untreated, the disease eventually moves into something called blast crisis, then advanced stage, then you're pretty much screwed (not a direct quote from Dr. Cathcart). Without treatment, CML typically kills patients within four to six years of diagnosis. Sheesh. I'd be 27, I thought. I just nodded and stared at Dr. Cathcart's ID badge. I could see that my mom's eyes were welling up with tears and I couldn't bear to look at her. Deep breath, I told myself.

Like most diseases, leukemia comes in many different forms. The more well-known are the acutes, particularly Acute Lymphocytic Leukemia, or ALL, which is often referred to as "childhood leukemia." The thing about ALL is that it's fast moving, so you have to be treated immediately. And you need heavy doses of chemo and radiation, which make you extremely ill. But, there is a more than 80 percent cure rate, a big light at the end of the tunnel. There's also a fast-moving myelogenous leukemia, AML, which, like ALL, is treated with chemo and radiation, but has a much lower cure rate—something like 30 percent. Then there's CLL, a slow-moving or chronic leukemia which, like CML, can be treated into deep remission but doesn't have a therapy as great as Gleevec and is difficult or impossible to cure. I was kind of hoping I'd have ALL, because of all the leukemias it has the highest cure rate and because I'd seen my friend beat it. To me, it seemed like if you had to have leukemia that was the one to get. But maybe I was wrong.

"What about this Gleevec thing?" my dad asked, his pen poised on a yellow legal pad. "That's the good news," Dr. Cathcart responded. In May 2001, six months before I was diagnosed, the FDA approved the breakthrough CML drug. It sailed through FDA trials faster than any other drug before it and was changing CML patients' lives, *saving* their lives. It was being called a miracle drug and was revolutionizing the way people looked at cancer. That's because Gleevec is a *pill*, a little orange pill that targets and kills only the cancer cells without harming healthy ones, which means there are relatively minor side effects—muscle cramping, heartburn and water retention are the most common (of course I'd get the one cancer that makes you fat, I thought). There's no hair loss, no vomiting, no greenish-gray skin—no need to get sick just to get well. "With Gleevec, patients can maintain a normal life," Dr. Cathcart said.

Having cancer and being normal didn't quite gel for me, but I went along with it. Dr. Cathcart said that with Gleevec I'd still be able to do everything I was doing before I was diagnosed: work out, eat sushi, take birth control, get manicures (my mom asked that one), go to work. "Drink?" I asked coyly—I was curious but didn't want to sound like a lush. Yes, she said. In moderation. In fact the *only* thing I couldn't do was eat grapefruit (something about it affecting the metabolism of the Gleevec). I was stunned. So was everyone else. My new life with cancer really could be just my old life with some pills thrown in.

"You're saying she could take a few pills, never feel sick, and be cured of a potentially deadly form of cancer without missing a day of work?" my dad asked.

"Not cured," Dr. Cathcart said. "But yes, she could do very well."

That was the catch. Gleevec was not a cure. When I was diagnosed, only about 50 percent of patients taking Gleevec had achieved remission but no one knew how long that remission would last. The longest anyone had been on the drug at that point was around two years, not enough time to gather much data on its long-term success. And no one who'd reached remission on the drug had ever stopped taking it—if they did, they'd likely relapse. Some miracle drug, I thought. If only 50 percent reached remission, what happened to the other half? Dr. Cathcart went on to say that the current statistics were based on the people in the original clinical trials. In order to take part in those trials, patients had to be very sick, so the results were based on people whose CML had been much more advanced than mine. One of the women in the *Glamour* story (which I had forced myself to read the night before) had been planning her funeral before she got the call that she'd been accepted into the trial. I was planning my 24th birthday party when I was diagnosed. Not exactly the same circumstances. But because I was in the early chronic phase, it was likely that I'd do considerably better than most. There were, of course, people for whom Gleevec didn't work at all. And there wasn't a lot of data on its long-term safety, either—I could grow a third arm for all they knew (though Dr. Cathcart assured me that that didn't seem likely). While Gleevec sounded better than the alternatives, I couldn't help having my doubts.

Dr. Cathcart asked if I had any siblings and I said yes, two sisters. That was good, she said. She wanted to have their blood tested to see if their bone marrow matched mine (each had a one in four chance). If the Gleevec didn't work, or if I relapsed down the road, having a transplant could save my life (or kill me, I thought). Because Gleevec was so new, there was a whole camp of doctors out there who were still recommending transplant as first-line treatment for young, otherwise healthy patients like me. Dr. Cathcart was not part of that camp, but she still thought my sisters should be tested right away. "A perfect match is like money in the bank," she said.

I made a mental note to start being nicer to Meghan, but I seriously doubted that either of my sisters would be my match. It seemed more likely that they'd match each other. For one, they looked a lot alike: They both had blue eyes, perfect noses and huge boobs (I have green eyes, a big nose and small boobs). Their personalities were much more similar, too. They were both really good at relaxing—they could sleep guilt-free till noon on a beautiful Saturday, then relocate to the couch and kill a bag of Ruffles while they watched *The Real World* marathon. If I slept past nine, I'd feel like I'd wasted the whole day. And I was more of a Baked Lays girl. Growing up they called themselves Bosom Buddies, a title Melissa got from the Tom Hanks sitcom of the same name. All it really meant was that Melissa could get Meghan to do whatever she wanted. "Go get me a glass of water or we won't be Bosom Buddies anymore," she'd say. And Meghan, who was six years younger, would do it. I was too smart to fall for Melissa's tricks, but that often meant that I got left out. I'd ask them if they wanted to play Barbies, and Melissa, who hated Barbies (the only way she'd ever play is if I let her be the hairdresser, which I couldn't always do because Barbie didn't need her hair done every single day) would say, "*Meggie?* Bosom Buddy? Did you forget you were going to watch me break my record on Frogger?" I just had a feeling that the same thing would happen with the bone marrow. I could already picture Melissa lying by my parents' pool telling Meghan to get her another margarita or they wouldn't be bone marrow buddies anymore.

"Do you have any questions?" Dr. Cathcart asked us. Mine was simple: I wanted to know if I was going to be OK, if I would survive all this. But I didn't ask it. I couldn't. Not in front of my parents. I didn't want them to know how scared I was. I had already perfected the "I'm going to be fine" attitude and I didn't want to let on that I wasn't quite so confident. My dad went first: "How did she get this?" he asked. "No one in our family has any kind of cancer," he added, sounding both proud and perplexed at the same time. Dr. Cathcart explained that they hadn't really pinpointed the exact cause of CML yet. Translation: They didn't have a clue how I got it. But it's not hereditary, she said. And it doesn't seem to be environmental, unless I was, in fact, living on a nuclear power plant. There is a higher rate of CML among people living in Hiroshima and Chernobyl, but Huntington was nothing like those places.

"The best way to explain it is that it's like being struck by lightning," Dr. Cathcart concluded. I loved this. I could live with being unlucky but I couldn't have handled it if she told me I had done something to bring it on myself. That was the whole reason I "quit" smoking pot after the first few times I tried it, and why I never once did a whippit or got on a motorcycle or had unprotected sex. I wanted to be good to my body so it would be good to me. I didn't want to do anything that might compromise my health in the future. Someone once told me I lived in a safety bubble, but I liked the way I lived. I was proud of everything I had done—and hadn't done. Sure I smoked a few cigarettes on spring break and raided my parents' liquor cabinet on occasion in high school, but that wasn't going to give me cancer. Relatively speaking, I was a good girl. And I really had no regrets (other than not becoming fluent in Spanish). Knowing that this CML garbage was unavoidable was such a relief, so oddly comforting. I had been struck by lightning—not pleasant, but not my fault. Fine by me. My father was less satisfied with that explanation and would spend the next several months coming up with different hypotheses to run by any doctor who would listen.

My mom's question was next: "How will all of this affect her fertility?" she asked. To my mom, having a family was the most important thing in life. And she was itching for some grandkids. "Because Gleevec is so new, they're not sure how it affects a developing fetus," Dr. Cathcart said. "so the drug company says not to take it if you are pregnant or think you may become pregnant." But, she assured us, that didn't mean I couldn't have children. It would just be complicated, something to discuss down the road. If I opted for a transplant, though, I would lose my fertility completely. I avoided looking at Nick. We weren't even sure we were going to get married and there we all were talking about our unborn babies. It was too much for me to think about. I would be lucky to have the dilemma of not being able to have children, I thought. That would mean that I was alive and well, maybe even cured.

Nick just sat there looking totally overwhelmed. I wondered if he was sorry he came to Sloan, or worse, to New York. Things had been going so well between us and now this. My mom later told me that she took Nick aside that morning and told him that it was going to be a long, tough journey and that if he wanted to leave, no one would think any less of him. He never mentioned that conversation to me, but I knew the thought of leaving had never occurred to him. It hadn't occurred to me either. In fact, I was a little insulted that my mom would even think there was a possibility he wouldn't stick around and I'm sure Nick was too. He loved me, and I loved him, and my getting cancer wasn't going to change that one bit.

"When can she start the Gleevec?" my dad asked, trying to shift the focus back to getting me well. I knew he wanted no part of the transplant, and neither did I. I could practically hear us saying, "Fuck that" in unison when Dr. Cathcart tossed out the 15 percent mortality rate. Gleevec was clearly my best option, but my white blood cell count was too high for me to start taking it yet. Dr. Cathcart wrote me a prescription for a drug called hydroxyurea, which she described as a Band-Aid—it would bring down my counts but it wouldn't do anything to stop the cancer. I'd get my blood checked once a week until my counts were normal. Then the Gleevec could go to work.

Before I left the hospital, I had to have a bone marrow biopsy, an excruciating procedure in which Dr. Cathcart screwed a six-inch-long needle into my hipbone near my lower back. Once the needle got past the bone, she sucked marrow out through the tiny hole in my back. It was very much like using a corkscrew to open a bottle of wine. I sneaked into the room alone, thank God, so no one else had to watch the torture. She also took a little piece of bone, which must have been the part when they told me I had to breathe (I'd bet they had people pass out on the table). That was the most excruciating pain I'd ever felt in my life. I was sweating right through my sweater. My hands clenched the sides of the table and I just cried and laughed and tried to remember to breathe. I thought a vein was going to pop out of my head, and the whole leukemia tragedy would be over because I'd be dead. The radio was playing some easy-listening song that kept repeating the line, "say it isn't so, say it isn't so." It made me smile. "What appropriate music," I said to Dr. Cathcart and the nurse who were busy cranking the needle deeper into my back. They chuckled politely, but quickly went back to business and I shut up. Making jokes always made me feel better in tough situations, like as long as we can still laugh, it can't be that bad. But it was.

I made an appointment to see Dr. Cathcart the following week and left with instructions to maintain a normal life. Whatever that was anymore, I thought. "So, um, should I be really worried?" I asked on my way out. So far I felt like I had a pretty good attitude, I said. But I wasn't sure if I was just kidding myself. "It's good to stay positive," she said. "It's good for your immune system." Huh? All I wanted to hear is that everything was going to be OK, but she couldn't tell me that, because she didn't know. No one did.

Now that I had the details, I had to get the word out. And I had to do it fast. I knew that once one person in Huntington found out, it wouldn't be long before it was the talk of the deli counter at King Kullen. And if I let the grapevine take care of it, they'd have me on my deathbed by the end of the week. I admit, it was pretty good gossip: "Did you hear about the Zammett girl? The one who works at *Glamour*, and lives in the city and has the seemingly perfect life? She has cancer. *Cancer.*" But it was *my* gossip, and I wanted to be the one to tell it. Plus, I wanted people to hear it from me so they knew I was OK, that I wasn't suddenly a leper who no one could touch or talk to. I made a million phone calls and sent an email to my crew of friends from high school: "I hope you're all sitting down," it began.

The phone didn't stop ringing. Even Alexis Fisher, a girl who I'd seen only once since she moved to Phoenix after the 9th grade, called to see how I was doing, to say she was thinking about me, praying for me. I was so grateful for the calls, and I knew they couldn't have been easy to make. I certainly wouldn't have wanted to talk to someone who'd just been diagnosed with cancer. What the hell do you say? I told the story over and over again. "Nope, no symptoms at all." "Yep, Gleevec. G.l.e.e.v.e.c." My mom was doing the same. At one point, I peeked over her shoulder while she was at the computer, emailing her friend Karen in Florida. "It's not the curable kind like Erik had," she wrote. "This is my worst nightmare. I wish it could be me." That made me cry. I felt so bad for my mom. She had already been through this once with me when I had ITP—she said the day they found out about that was the scariest moment of her life.

My best friend, Erin, and I had just walked home from art class and were headed up to the pool to play sharks and minnows. My mom stopped me when she saw bruises and little red dots all over my legs. She called the pediatrician who told her to bring me in right away. He took some blood and sent me home, saying he'd call as soon as he had the results. Minutes after we arrived back home, the doctor called. "Where's Erin?" he asked. "On the swing set playing," my mom said. The doctor told her to put down the phone, go get me, sit me down and not let me move. My platelet count was dangerously low, and he didn't want me banging my head and bleeding to death (the red dots on my legs meant I was already bleeding under the skin). When my mom got back to the phone, the doctor told her to drive me straight to Schneider Children's Hospital. He was pretty sure I had leukemia.

After a round of tests—including a bone marrow biopsy that I no longer remember—they figured out that it was not, in fact, leukemia, but a much less scary, much more easily treatable, disease. (No wonder doctors don't speculate anymore.) Still, I was admitted and my mom spent two weeks sleeping next to me in a chair. On the cancer ward no less. She had to watch her little third-grader get blood tests and platelet transfusions and even worse, play with my new friends—really sick kids with little hair and less hope, who'd skate around happily on their IV poles when they weren't throwing up from all the chemo. For me, it wasn't so bad. In fact, other than the needles in the arm, I had a blast. I was on prednisone, a steroid that increases your appetite, so I was constantly eating, which had always been my favorite thing to do anyway. My dad would bring me Burger King and Chinese takeout and calzones from Junior's Pizzaria (no beef stroganoff, thank you very much). The hospital food wasn't too bad either. I got three little menus every night to order what I wanted to eat the next day. I always put two check marks and wrote "extra crispy" next to the bacon on the breakfast menu. That was my all-time favorite food. I got lots of presents while I was there too, including the very popular, though previously too expensive to buy for me, Benetton Bear (in green). And Walkie Talkies, which made me the coolest kid on the floor. I also had my mom's undivided attention, which was very hard to come by, but very lovely when you had it. She later told me that she prayed to God every single night we were there and said that she would never yell at me again if I just got better. Well I did get better and she did yell at me again. But I'm sure I deserved it.

As much as I dreaded it, I really needed to tell Meghan about my leukemia. I was starting to fear that she might hear it through the grapevine, which incidentally did run all the way to Tennessee. When I called, her roommate had to get her out of bed (it was 11 a.m. on a Friday) and before I could even say hello she started telling me about the horrible nightmares she'd had all night. Earthquakes and shaking. She hadn't slept a wink. "Wow, Meg, that sucks. So I have some good news and I have some bad news," I said, trying to launch right into my spiel and get it over with. "The good news is I'll be home for Thanksgiving," I said. Nick and I had been planning to go to Flint, Michigan, to spend the holiday with his family, but cancer changed our plans. I was secretly thrilled we weren't going. Holidays were big productions in my family and though they were inevitably stressful, they were also inevitably fun. Not to mention, you were kind of a shit if you didn't show. Meghan got all excited, but then asked why I wasn't going to Michigan. "Well, that's the bad news," I said and told her I got some blood tests back and as it turns out I have a little blood disease but I'm perfectly fine. She asked what kind of disease it was and I said, "You know." I just couldn't bear to say the word. "Think about it. You know. What do you think it is?" I asked, actually making her guess. "TB?" she said. "No Meg," I said, "Not tuberculosis." (Later, she told me that she meant ITP, not TB.) Then she said, "Like what, Er?" And I said, "Like leukemia, Meg, cancer. But I'm fine and it's no big deal." She pretty much lost it. There's really no sugarcoating cancer.

Having Thanksgiving fall a week into my diagnosis worked out well. I could let everyone see for themselves that I was OK. We always have Thanksgiving dinner with my father's side of the family at my Aunt Donna and Uncle Neil's house. They live a few towns over from Huntington. With all the cousins and cousins' kids and girlfriends and great uncles, there are usually 30 people gathered around the table (actually the four tables Aunt Donna has to push together to accommodate all of us). Needless to say, I was a bit anxious. Aunt Donna had called me a few days earlier and asked me if I wanted to say grace. Yikes, I thought. With Grandma Ruth's health on the fritz (she'd practically had a stroke at the table the year before) and Uncle Mike's epic war stories and Aunt Betsy showing up late every year, there would be enough melodrama without the newly appointed leukemia patient saying a prayer. People would be sad enough just watching me eat my turkey. "But she looks so good, how can it be?" I told Aunt Donna thanks, but I'd rather wait and say it in five years or so when I'm cancer free. Then it would be appropriate. Aunt Donna takes her holidays very seriously—she starts setting the Thanksgiving table a week early to make sure everything is perfect—and she lives to make people happy. She just thought saying grace would make me feel special, be a nice touch for Thanksgiving '01. When I told my mom about Aunt Donna's request she said, "Jesus Christ, is she trying to kill me?"

As it turned out, there was no drama at all. My oldest cousin, Beth, said a lovely grace, and we all ate our turkey and mashed potatoes like good little pilgrims. It was clear that everyone was on their best behavior. Grandma Ruth was pleasant and stroke free, Uncle Mike, who was 88, sliced the turkey like a champ, and no one got too drunk. My Aunt Kathie had had skin cancer removed from her nose the day before, and looked like she'd been beaten up, so no one paid much attention to me at all. Grandma Del, my mom's mom, did corner me at one point, though. She had seen Nick and me standing very close and swooped in to make sure we weren't too "serious" or doing anything "stupid." I guess she meant marriage, though come to think of it she probably meant sex—too late. Even at 79, my grandma was spunky, and a huge flirt. She just thought I should be playing the field. (It still hadn't occurred to her that two and half years with Nick meant we were serious.) Thank God I didn't have to play the field. I couldn't even imagine having to tell some guy in a bar that I had leukemia. That doesn't exactly make me a catch. "I like reading and sports and long walks at sunset. And oh yeah, I have cancer and I may die." Thank God for Nick. I knew it wasn't easy for him, but he was handling everything so well, mostly just by being himself and keeping me smiling. When we were getting ready to head to Aunt Donna's and I was stressing about my outfit—for a change—he said, "You look beautiful. If there was a Miss Leukemia Pageant, you'd win hands down."

We did have our sad moments, though. Earlier that day I'd been lying on my bed at my parents' house trying to rest a bit and Nick came into the bedroom. He pointed to a little picture frame on a shelf above my bed and said, "Aww." He grabbed it to show to me, but I already knew what he was talking about. It was a picture of me on Halloween when I was 5. I was dressed as a fat little bumblebee with a curly black wig. I had an embarrassed look on my face, with my hands behind my little bee wings. It was so cute, but it made us both cry. I looked so sweet and innocent in that picture, my whole bee life was ahead of me. Now I was 23 and I had cancer. Our faces were soaked with tears. Then I told him that my friend Erin's older sister nicknamed me bumble-butt after seeing me in that costume—and called me that until I was about 10. Then we started laughing.

A few days after Thanksgiving, Dr. Cathcart called to give me the results of my biopsy. She told me it all checked out as expected: I was in chronic phase and there were no crazy mutations. I officially, 100 percent, had CML. The regular kind. While I had her on the phone, I figured I'd feel her out, see if she felt like throwing me a bone this time, telling me I was going to live. I told her that all my friends and family couldn't believe how well I was handling everything and that that was starting to scare me, like maybe they knew something I didn't. She just repeated the line about how keeping a positive attitude was good for me. And that I had reason to be hopeful. I liked Dr. Cathcart, but the whole vague doctor thing was beginning to get to me. Couldn't she shoot me straight? Even if I were going to die, I'd rather she just tell me. I hated not knowing what was going to happen.

I began to wonder if I should run to church and start praying. It seemed like the right thing to do, but I didn't want to be one of those people who gets sick and suddenly finds God. I grew up Catholic, but my churchgoing had lapsed in the last few years and I felt like God would be thinking "sure, you're here now but where were you when everything was good in your life, huh?" My mom, who had always been a good Catholic girl, brought my sisters and me to church every single Sunday when we were little. My father, who had gone to Catholic school his whole life, was an altar boy for years and could recite obscure passages out of the Bible, was a devout atheist. He didn't even go to our baptisms (he had made a deal with my mom that if he got married in the church, he'd never have to step foot in one again). He's lightened up over the years and now attends weddings and funerals of people he really likes/liked. Anyway, when we got into high school, my mom gave up on forcing us to go to church and we devolved into Easter and Christmas Catholics.

There were a few months during my senior year of college when I decided that Nick and I should start going to church together. We went every Sunday for two months, but I had to bribe him with sex, which made me feel guilty before I even got there.

My godfather, Steve, one of my father's oldest friends (and a serious Catholic), told me that I shouldn't be worried about whether or not I'd been to church in the past six months because "God is with you." Hearing him say that made me cry, but pretty much any nice thing people said to me was making me cry. I decided I would start small and light a candle for myself at St. Patrick's Cathedral one day after work. It seemed kind of like throwing your own surprise birthday party, but I figured I could really use it.

Meanwhile, I had my first sign that there was actually something wrong with me. It was just a little rash from the hydroxyurea, not the cancer, but still, it somehow made me feel better, proof that this wasn't all some big hoax. I also started getting a little nauseated when I first took my dose, but I was OK with that, too. It made sense to me. Cancer *should* suck. Or at the very least be a drag. At least with some side effects, I had something tangible to complain about (other than having to give up grapefruit, of course). I could start believing that all of this was really happening.

While we were waiting for my counts to normalize, I decided to call Brian Druker, the doctor who headed up the development of Gleevec and was featured in the *Glamour* story. He was based at a hospital called Oregon Health and Sciences University in Portland, Oregon. Though I felt like I was in good hands with Dr. Cathcart, I figured it couldn't hurt to make the contact, see if he had any insight to offer me. I spoke with his assistant, a girl who couldn't have been any older than me, which somehow made me sad. She sounded healthy, why couldn't I be healthy? I told her I was from *Glamour*. She remembered the article and was happy to set up an informational meeting with Dr. Druker. I hadn't thought about going all the way across the country to meet him, but it seemed like a decent idea. She also told me about some clinical trials that OHSU was planning. Though Gleevec's success was making headlines, Dr. Druker and his team were already looking for ways to make it more efficient for newly diagnosed patients. The trials would combine Gleevec with injections of low-dose chemotherapy, which the doctors believed would work like a one-two punch. Having already gotten used to the pill-popping/normal life idea, I wasn't totally psyched about this discovery. Mostly because I knew I'd wind up doing it. If there were some way to make me better, faster, then I needed to be a part of it, even if it meant stabbing myself with needles. They'd have to do some tests to see if I was eligible, which Kelly said they could take care of when I came out to meet Dr. Druker. I told her I'd run everything by my parents and call her back.

Despite my earlier concern about being able to drink, I still hadn't had any alcohol since I was diagnosed. I just didn't feel like it. (My mom got me non-alcoholic wine for Thanksgiving, which was a nice gesture, but totally disgusting.) So far I felt pretty good, and I didn't want to screw that up. I wanted to do everything I could to make my body 100 percent, or as close to 100 percent as a cancer patient could get. I stressed less and slept more. And I ate more, too—I had always had a healthy, well-balanced diet, but I loosened it up a bit. I let myself eat Ben & Jerry's, which I rationalized as calcium, and bacon, egg and cheese sandwiches (protein) and I started eating more red meat (iron). But I made sure I was working out enough, too. As crazy as it may sound, I knew that if I started to gain weight, I would get more depressed about that than the cancer. Despite my whirlwind diagnosis, I was still 23, living in New York City and working at a flashy magazine. Looking good had always been important to me and that wasn't going to change. Even when we left Sloan after my biopsy that first day, I went straight to

Bloomie Nails with my mom for an eyebrow wax. "Is this weird?" I asked her when we walked in. Maybe we should be home, under the covers, crying, I thought. Isn't that what people who just found out they have cancer do? "Not if you need an eyebrow wax," my mom said. And I did. And we were in the neighborhood.

In some ways I think I felt like if I kept my body in shape, if I kept looking good, the cancer would get confused and leave. Or at the very least people wouldn't pity me, whisper at their cubicles about sad, sickly Erin. I did realize that I was lucky to be able to worry about admittedly silly things like eyebrows and two pounds, lucky to be at my desk every day instead of some hospital bed wasting away. I just didn't want that luck to run out.

3 There must be some kind of mistake

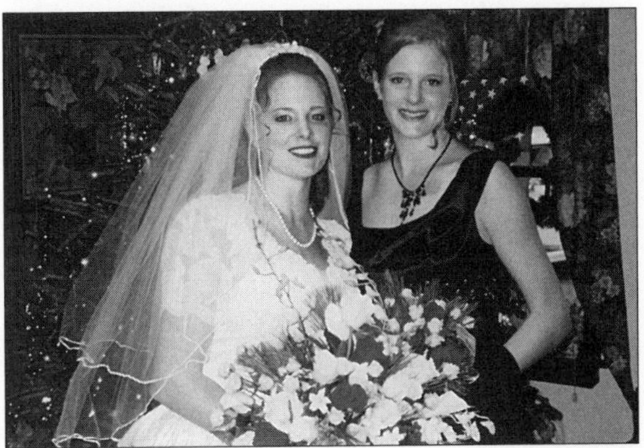

With my sister, Melissa, on her wedding day

IF THERE WERE EVER SOMETHING THAT COULD STEAL Melissa's wedding-day thunder, it was my being diagnosed with leukemia six weeks before her big day. Just like that, the happiest time of her life was eclipsed by the worst time of mine. My mom traded in dress-fitting and menu tasting appointments with Melissa for trips to Sloan with me. We tried to act interested in her bride-to-be dilemmas, but which type of oyster to serve at the cocktail hour, and whether the bridesmaids' toenail polish should match their fingernail polish just didn't seem that important anymore. In some ways, though, my cancer was the best thing to happen to Melissa's wedding. My mom became so distracted by everything going on with me that she started saying yes to all of Melissa's costly requests, signing checks without question. Chamber ensemble to play outside the church? Sure. Excaliber to drive you the .2 miles from the church to the reception? What the hell! "It's only money" became my mom's favorite saying. And Melissa happily cashed in.

Melissa told me that when I was first diagnosed, she felt so bad for me that she immediately wished it were her. Then she quickly changed her mind when she realized I was much better equipped for a disease than she was (and that she didn't want to have leukemia on her wedding day). Melissa was a serious hypochondriac—always dying of some strange disease or another—so she figured it would have been pretty bad if she actually did have something wrong with her. She said she would have quit her job and moved back in with my parents and started eating every meal like it was her last. The remote control would have become her best friend. She just knew that I would handle it better than she ever could. I heard that from a lot of people. If anyone had to get cancer, it *should* be me because I'd be the one to beat it. And they all said I'd make something good come out of it too. It was oddly flattering to know that people had that much confidence in me to be so sure I'd overcome cancer. But I also felt a little pressure. I couldn't let everyone down.

A few weeks after I was diagnosed, Cindi, *Glamour*'s editor-in-chief, dropped by my desk to see if I'd be interested in writing about my experience for the magazine. I had secretly been hoping she'd ask, but we had just done the feature on those three women with CML so I figured my story was old news. "I think our readers would be intensely interested in getting to know a young cancer patient," she said, "your thoughts and fears." She said maybe we'd make it a recurring column where readers could follow my progress. I tried to hide my excitement—the editor-in-chief was asking me to write about my life in her magazine!—and told her I'd been keeping a detailed journal and would love to share it.

Right before I was diagnosed, my parents had given me a gorgeous leather-bound journal—it was green with a half-dollar size piece of Murano glass in the cover. They had brought it back from Venice for me, and I'd been struggling to come up with something worthy to fill its pages. I had always documented the major moments in my life—I have Ronald McDonald spiral notebooks filled with giant lettering from when I was five: "We R at Disney Wrld with Grammy Ruth. It is rely fun. Goofy is my favrite." But I couldn't bear to relive September 11, and my daily struggles—being overworked and underpaid, needing a new hairstyle, my roommate leaving every single cabinet in our kitchen open—weren't interesting enough to chronicle. Now, suddenly, I had all the material I'd ever need. I started scribbling down everything, almost as it was happening. I didn't go anywhere without my journal. And though it was tough to put it all in words sometimes, I knew that, ultimately, writing about my experience would make living it that much easier. Cindi said to keep writing and we'd talk soon.

The week before Christmas, my parents and I flew out to Oregon to meet Dr. Druker and his colleague, Dr. Michael Mauro, the guy who was heading up the new clinical trials. When Donald, whose desk was about half a foot away from mine, heard about the trip, he said he was sending a camera crew. If I was going to be writing about my experience for the magazine, then he needed photos to go with it. From here on out, he had to know about every important event in my life so he could shoot it. Sounds good to me, I thought. It would be like having my very own cancer paparazzi. Plus, I was really nervous about going to Oregon so having photographers in tow would be a good distraction, make me feel like it was just some elaborate photo shoot. I certainly didn't look the part of patient, and I didn't feel it, so why should I have to play it? As I was leaving the office to go to the airport, Donald called down the hallway to me, "Remember to cry!" I loved him for that.

On the plane, I was wedged in the middle seat between my mother and my father, like a little kid who had done something bad. Unable to get a good view of the in-flight movie, I started reading a pamphlet on CML that Dr. Cathcart had given me the day we met. So far, I had avoided reading much on the subject—too depressing—but I figured I should brush up so as not to embarrass myself in front of the pros. I mean what kind of patient doesn't even know what the *M* in their CML means? The paragraph on survival statistics jumped out at me immediately. As I read it, tears just started rolling down my face. Though I really had adjusted to having cancer, there were still moments when that new reality would hit hard. For all of us. Like when my dad rode the Long Island Railroad with Melissa's blood sitting next to him in a little cooler. Dr. Cathcart had given us blood collection kits so that my sisters wouldn't have to make special trips into the city to find out if they were bone marrow matches for me. They could get their blood drawn at a local clinic and then FedEx it back to Sloan for testing. Melissa had hers done at Huntington Hospital and my dad, who was going into the city the next day for a business meeting, offered to drop it off at Sloan. Big mistake. He later told me that sitting on the train reading *Theodore Rex* with his daughter's blood on his lap—hoping that it might someday be able to save the life of his other daughter—was one of the saddest, most surreal moments of his life.

For me, many of those moments came at work. I'd be in the middle of editing a page on "Guys' Biggest Under-the-Cover Regrets" and have to stop what I was doing to go to Sloan for a 3 p.m. checkup. Boom—back to finger sticks and blood counts. And while spending an afternoon in a waiting room full of cancer patients did give me some perspective on my deadline anxieties, I always left feeling totally depressed. In the beginning, especially, it was a bit of a roller coaster ride. Some days I felt nothing. I couldn't make myself cry if I wanted to. Even if I said in my head over and over again, "you could die from this, this is very bad, you have cancer" it didn't register, like I was in some kind of calm coma, numb to the whole thing. I worried that maybe I was in denial, that I wasn't fully comprehending the gravity of my disease, not taking it seriously enough. Then other days, I wouldn't be able to focus because my head would be overflowing with cancer thoughts: Would I live to be 30? Would I ever be cured? Would I be able to have kids? On those days if someone smiled at me on the street, I would cry.

It was raining when we got to Portland, which I soon learned was to be expected. Still, I immediately loved the city. With its rivers and bridges, it reminded me of Knoxville, only bigger and with less traffic. There were trolleys and cobblestone streets and water fountains on every corner. There was also a Saks and a Nordstroms and no sales tax—though, as my dad reminded us, we weren't there to shop.

First on our agenda was a meeting with Dr. Mauro, a short, thin 30-something guy with blue-tinted glasses and a gentle voice. I liked him immediately. He was from Long Island—bonus points—and had trained alongside Dr. Cathcart in New York City, which would prove to be a very handy coincidence. Our meeting was informative, but all the medical talk was a little snooze-inducing. It was kind of like being in science class—except now my life depended on getting an A; back in high school I only *thought* it did. He told us about the two trials they were conducting—one combined Gleevec with injections of Interferon; the other combined Gleevec with injections of Ara-C. (Interferon and Ara-C were the two drugs used to treat CML before Gleevec was developed.) The idea behind the combination was that any leukemia cells not destroyed by the Gleevec would be picked up by the other drug. Recalling from the *Glamour* article that the side effects of the injections weren't pretty, I asked Dr. Mauro to elaborate—honestly. Well, he said, the Interferon could cause nausea, fatigue and depression; the Ara-C could cause nausea, fatigue and dangerously low blood counts. But, he assured us, the doses for the trial were so low that any side effects I did experience could easily be managed with drugs. I hated the idea of having to treat the side effects of drugs with more drugs. Just a month ago I'd been a girl who would't even take Advil.

Both trials would require me to spend a considerable amount of time in Portland—two weeks initially to get started, then a visit at least every three months for the year-long duration. I could hear the dollar signs adding up in my father's head. My parents had plenty of money, but my dad didn't always love to spend it. He would take us on great vacations and treat his friends to expensive dinners but never hire a plumber to fix a toilet, or call information for a phone number or spend more than $30 on a pair of pants. My equally frugal mom was consistently appalled by her daughters' flip attitude about money. "$60 for a haircut? You must be very rich," she'd say. (Unisex Palace, the place she had always taken us as kids, made SuperCuts look like Oscar Blandi.) My parents had worked their asses off to get where they were—and they weren't going to blow that on a jumbo popcorn when you could just as easily pop your own and sneak it into the theater (something my mom actually made us do when we were little). But I knew cancer was different. My mom later told me that they had already talked about selling the house if it came to that. They would do anything if it meant getting me well.

Because I hadn't started any real treatment yet—and other than having cancer I was perfectly healthy—I was eligible for either trial. It sounded to me like the Interferon combination was the more hard-core of the two, so I assumed that one would yield the best results. I asked Dr. Mauro if he agreed. "Well, I can't really say which one is better," he replied. God I hated the non-answer answer. "I can't really tell you what to do." He was incredibly nice about dodging my questions and he would soon become one of my favorite people in the whole world, but right then I wanted to shake him. Wasn't that why I came all the way to freakin' Oregon? I knew nothing about anything—even after reading my CML brochure I still couldn't tell you what the M meant—how the hell was I supposed to make that call on my own? I couldn't even pick out a movie at Blockbuster without having a near-anxiety attack or order dinner without changing my mind three times and still end up wishing I had gotten something else. I couldn't make a decision to save my life. And now that was exactly what I had to do.

But not yet. Apparently the FDA makes you jump through hoops when you want to experiment on patients and even the smallest typo on a hospital's application form can stall the approval process for weeks. In other words, neither trial was starting yet. Dr. Mauro assured us that they would be green-lighted soon, though. In the meantime, I should continue to take the hydroxurea. I couldn't help thinking that it was a little strange for these doctors to allow my CML to go untreated. It had been over a month since I was diagnosed. Wasn't the cancer progressing? Shouldn't I be doing something to stop it?

Dr. Mauro gave me a quick exam and asked me a bunch of questions about my health: Did I have night sweats? Chills? Headaches? Chest pains? Shortness of breath? I answered no over and over. "I feel perfectly healthy," I said. It was my canned response, but saying it to the doctor made me feel like it was true. Like maybe he'd just take my word for it and send me home, tell me there must be some kind of mistake. "Come to think of it, you don't have leukemia at all," he'd say. "So sorry to make you come all the way out to Oregon just to send you home. Merry Christmas." Of course that didn't happen. My bad blood betrayed me.

The *Glamour* photographers snapped shots the whole time we were there, which made everything feel a little staged. I was more concerned with how my hair was going to look in the photos than with the discussion of my long-term survival rates. I sucked in my stomach the whole time and even grabbed a tissue at one point to pretend blot my eyes for the camera. I was too detached from what was going on to actually cry about it, but I adored Donald and desperately wanted to please him. So I faked it. Before we left, the photographer said he wanted to get a shot of a group hug. My family doesn't do group hugs, but we figured what the hell. When in Cancerland . . . The photo ran in the magazine with my first column and though I looked like I was burying my head in my mom's shoulder, crying, I was actually laughing hysterically at how silly I felt (not that I admitted this to anyone back at *Glamour*).

After our photo shoot—I mean cancer meeting—we headed down to the research building where we were introduced to Dr. Druker. He was very tall and very thin, with very twinkling eyes, almost like he was up to something. He was my first cancer celebrity, and I was a little nervous to be talking to him. This guy had even been in *Glamour*! His brain probably carried the cure for cancer, but his office was a bit of a hole in the wall. Couldn't they give him a few plants? I thought. Maybe a window? We asked Dr. Druker a few general leukemia questions, and he gave us a straight answer every time, with no medical jargon and none of the doctorly vagueness I'd come to expect. Then I asked what he thought I should do. "If I were you," he said, "I'd go with the Gleevec/Interferon trial." I loved him for giving us his opinion. Then he added, "unless I had a perfect match for a transplant." What?! This was the man who practically invented Gleevec, and he's saying he wouldn't necessarily take it? He said that because I was so young, I could do very well with a transplant and be completely cured and that it was something to consider. But we still hadn't heard about my sisters' blood, so there was no use talking about it further. I returned to New York with more questions than answers.

Meanwhile, Santa Claus was coming to town. I don't think anyone was prepared, or necessarily in the spirit, but we went through the motions anyway. My mom had turned the house into the usual winter wonderland, complete with tiny ice skaters who actually skate through a hand-painted Christmas village, so we had no choice but to be jolly. Every year on Christmas Eve, we have a party at my parents' house and despite September 11 and cancer at 23, the show had to go on. It's always a casual night—people stop by before midnight mass, or after their own Christmas Eve dinners, my dad makes his famous, lethal, hot apple cider, we put out some clam dip, hang the mistletoe and mingle. Then, at midnight, Melissa, Meghan and I sit in front of the fireplace and read *'Twas the Night before Christmas.* We've done this every Christmas Eve for as long as I can remember. It was probably adorable when three little redheaded girls sat up there in their fuzzies, but lately it had been three *big* redheaded girls who had had a little too much of Daddy's cider. Not as cute, but still a good time. Meghan always got nervous and stumbled over her words and Melissa would crack up then direct the spotlight back to her—"on Dancer, on Prancer, on Comet and Vixen," she'd say with one hand slightly raised as if she were reading a Shakespeare soliloquy. Whichever one of us wound up getting the last page and reading the line, "Merry Christmas to all, and to all a good night" was the envy of the other two. We all wanted the big finish. Our guests—most of whom counted on this little display as part of their own Christmas tradition—would clap and cheer and raise a glass. Then my mom would kick everyone out so Santa Claus could do her job.

This year, an unusually large number of my friends showed up. It was nice to see them, of course, but as I looked around at faces I hadn't seen in months, it got me thinking. I was *that girl*, the one who people felt bad for, and prayed for and thanked God they were not. It was a sad realization. I had always thought of myself as someone people looked up to, someone people wanted to be like. But I was no longer enviable. I was pitied. I was that person from your high school that your mom told you about when you came home for the holidays.

"Oh honey did you hear about Erin Zammett?"

"Yeah, that totally sucks. I heard she found out at just, like, a normal checkup. So, what's for dinner, Mom?"

Huntington has a population of almost 200,000, but everyone knows everyone else's business. And there was always one sad story making the rounds—a terrible car accident, an ugly divorce, a cancer diagnosis. I just couldn't get over the fact that the sad story was mine. And I worried that people didn't have that story straight as they traded their gossip at the nail salon or the car wash. Tricia, a longtime friend, called me the day after I was diagnosed and said she heard that the doctor thought I was pregnant at first. Huh? At least that one was harmless. My old boyfriend also called and told me that he had gotten an email from a girl we went to high school with that read, "I heard Erin Zammett has leukemia and is dying." First, I couldn't believe that he would call me up to tell me that—did it not occur to him that I *did* have leukemia and maybe I didn't want to know that people thought I had one foot in the grave? Then I wondered where that girl got the information and how many other people she had emailed. It pissed me off, but more than that, it upset me. To hear that other people were talking about my leukemia made it real somehow, and made me feel like maybe it was true, that I *was* dying and I was the only idiot who hadn't gotten the memo. That had always been my biggest pet peeve—other people knowing something about me that I didn't know. Like when the boy I dated for about a week in junior high wanted to break up with me and the whole eighth grade heard about it before I did. Nothing made me feel more stupid. And this was a little more serious than being dumped by a kid who was too short for me and last I heard wound up in jail for selling crack. I didn't want people to think I was dying. Because I wasn't and I had no plans to either.

Christmas morning was the usual scene. My sisters and I wore matching pajamas—which my mom gives us every year—and our Santa hats with our names glittered on them. Ysrael had one, too. We posed for silly pictures while the dogs tore through packages of candycane-shaped bones, and my dad sat in the La-Z-Boy in the corner, pretending to be interested in every pair of socks and box of golf balls he opened. "Just what I needed," he'd say, sometimes sincerely, sometimes sarcastically. He didn't like Christmas very much and usually had at least one major blow-up a season. I was never sure if he was so stressed because he was adding up my mother's excessive expenditures present by present, or because he had such bad memories of Christmases growing up. His family wasn't exactly the Brady Bunch. He learned to drive when he was 14 mostly so that when he got calls from the VFW to pick up his drunken dad, he could keep it from his mom. He'd ride down to the bar on his bike, throw it—and his dad—into his dad's car, jump in the driver's seat and make his way home. Then his mom would scream at him for protecting his father.

They had a tumultuous relationship, but I knew my dad loved his father—and missed him very much. One Christmas when I was about 12 my mom sent me down to the basement to get some eggs out of the spare refrigerator and I saw my dad standing in front of his workbench staring at something. I asked him what he was doing. "Just wishing my father a Merry Christmas," he said. He was looking up at a dusty old sketch of his father that hung above the bench. I backed away, went up to my bedroom and started crying. My dad's father (I never knew him, so I never felt comfortable calling him Grampy, like some of my older cousins did) died in a plane crash when he was 53. He was a commercial pilot for Pan Am, but that day he was flying a cargo plane to Prestwick, Scotland. He liked flying cargo and had done that route so many times that he had a regular golf lesson with a pro in Prestwick. The cargo (chemicals that were going to a semi-conductor plant in Scotland) had been packed wrong and burst into flames while they were somewhere in the middle of the Atlantic Ocean. He turned the plane around in an attempt to land it at Logan Airport in Boston but the smoke was too much and the three-man crew suffocated before they made it. Witnesses said they saw heads sticking out of the window, apparently gasping for air, before the plane hit just shy of runway 27. It happened about a month before Christmas. Because my father was an air-traffic controller at the time, he heard about the crash over the radios almost immediately. Then he had to go identify the body. He was 29. That story, which my dad only ever told me once, haunted me throughout my childhood. I could only imagine what it did to him. If he was a Scrooge around the holidays, there was good reason for it.

My mom went completely overboard on gifts for Ysrael. It was his first Christmas with the family and she really wanted him to feel welcome. Plus he'd grown up with nothing in a place where they glue wine corks to the bottom of their sneakers to make soccer cleats. She couldn't help but spoil him. Seeing how happy he was—and how happy Melissa was—made me feel guilty for ever questioning their relationship. Before I was diagnosed all any of us could talk about was why Melissa was marrying a guy who barely spoke English. Now it was almost embarrassing that we were all worked up over something so minor. So what if he's a little different, he loves her and she's happy—and healthy.

Having Ysrael around for Christmas made me miss Nick, who had gone back to Michigan for a few days to be with his family. We had been getting along really well lately. And we had finally broken our cancer celibacy, too, which wasn't nearly as weird as I thought it would be. Nick was like my best friend, my boyfriend and my brother all rolled into one (brother only because he was living with my parents). I felt a little lost without him around. He was the one person I could really talk to about everything going on in my head, my doubts and fears. My family only addressed my cancer in practical terms. They wanted to know if I took my medicine or if the doctor called with any news on the trial. They didn't want to know that I lay awake at night sometimes crying, scared to death that this was happening to me. I knew that my illness was their number one priority, hands down, but they weren't good at talking about it. My mom just cried, and that killed me, and my dad would bring up his new Italian barstools or the score of the Jets game. If I tried to talk to Melissa, she would just say, "Er, you're going to be fine, look at you!" It's not that I was trying to turn my family into a big depressing support group, but sometimes I just wanted to talk about how crazy it was that I had cancer.

Nick and I called each other about seven times a day while he was gone. Mostly, we talked about what was going on at the other person's house: lots at mine; nothing at his. Growing up, Nicky didn't have to do anything Nicky didn't want to do. He was spoiled, even though his parents didn't have much money. This made his upbringing very different from mine, and caused more than a few clashes in our relationship. And when he went home, which was rare, the same rule applied. So while I was cleaning up the living room and helping my mom prepare dinner, Nick was lying on the couch watching *It's a Wonderful Life* in between naps. But I was glad he was getting a chance to relax, especially since the whole Nicky only does what Nicky wants to do rule didn't apply in New York. And even just hearing his voice for a minute made me feel better.

We got the news that Melissa's marrow didn't match mine two days after Christmas. I was sitting at my desk at work when Dr. Cathcart called. She was only a half match, which was completely useless to me. (It would be like driving over half a bridge; not exactly a good route to take.) I was disappointed, but prepared. I didn't even get that upset—but then, how could I fully understand the importance? I was eating a yogurt parfait and

RSVPing to my friend Ali's art gallery opening e-vite at the time. Not exactly dire circumstances. Despite what my blood tests showed, I still felt fine, so it was hard to imagine a day when I'd be lying in a hospital bed, praying for a last chance at life. But it was a definite possibility.

Now Meghan was my only hope, but her results wouldn't be back for a few weeks. She hadn't gotten her blood drawn in Knoxville like she was supposed to—she claimed that she never knew that was the plan—so she didn't get to do it until the week before Christmas when she arrived home for break, which really pissed me off. I decided I'd take her in to Sloan myself—a very bad idea. We were at my parents' house and we were running late for the train. Meghan was upstairs putting on her makeup—she wouldn't go anywhere without looking perfect, a process that took time and precision and was a major point of contention between us. I paced around downstairs, desperately trying not to freak out.

Nothing got me more worked up than running late, but somehow I was always running late. I had been known to get so angry that I'd punch walls and slam doors and throw things. (I never did this at work or in front of my friends; only in front of my family, which I realize didn't make it right.) I definitely had issues with rage, and I was planning to work them out eventually, maybe even see a therapist. Then I found out I had cancer and figured I had bigger fish to fry. And being diagnosed calmed me down immediately—but that serenity didn't last long.

"Drop the fucking mascara and get your ass down here," I screamed up the stairs. "I'll be in the car."

I walked outside and slammed the door as hard as I could. That was only the beginning. By the time Meghan walked outside, slowly and looking clueless, I was screaming. "Are you serious??!! We're going to miss the fucking train, Goddamn it!" And then I heaved my banana into the woods and smashed my cup of water into the driveway. I was fuming. My face was bright red and I really felt like I could have killed her.

My mom, who was driving us to the train station, started yelling at me to calm down, which only made me more angry.

"Calm down? Calm down? We're going to miss the fucking train and by the time we get to Sloan we're going to have to wait forever and then I'm going to be so late for work that I may as well not even go!"

Then I smashed my elbow into the side of the car and screamed. So much for the even-keeled cancer patient I thought I had become. When my mom threatened to drop me off at 5 North—the nuthouse at Huntington Hospital—instead of the train station, I began to calm down. Then I started crying. Whenever I got that mad, I immediately felt guilty. I'd spend days feeling like a shit, beating myself up, wishing I could control my anger, wishing I wasn't such a freak. And being a cancer patient made that process even worse. How could I get that upset about missing a train when I have this disease to contend with? And how could I be so mean to Meghan? I needed her. I just knew that I had blown any chance I had that she would be my match. God would definitely punish me for being such an asshole.

I also felt like I had failed the disease in some way, failed to have that newfound perspective on life that I thought came with every diagnosis. Surely cancer patients weren't supposed to throw bananas and scream at their sisters. I should be kind and good and just happy to be alive. But, slowly, the old me was creeping back in and I couldn't stop it. That was the worst day I'd had since I was diagnosed.

New Year's came and went without incident—and without resolutions (except to try to be less of a psycho). I just didn't think I needed to give anything up. I had cancer, wasn't that enough of a sacrifice? And it didn't seem like the year to make a fresh start with something, finally get my photo albums organized, or get painting again. It seemed strange to be toasting to health and happiness. I felt like saying, let's be honest here—health and happiness? I don't think so. There was really no time to ponder life, though, surprise, surprise. Melissa and Ysrael's wedding was on January 4th and the troops started rolling in early. For the next five days, chaos would reign.

Since we had a ton of cousins in town, Dr. Cathcart said we should bring them to Sloan to have their blood tested, too. It was unlikely that any of their bone marrows would match mine, but it couldn't hurt to try. Jessica and Lauren, my southern belle cousins, were first. My Uncle B.J. and Aunt Mary brought them to Sloan directly from the airport. But it didn't go so well. The phlebotomist couldn't find a vein in Lauren, the 11-year-old, and while they were hunting for one, Jessica, the 14-year-old who was watching, got freaked out and started crying. Seeing her big sister cry made Lauren upset so she started crying, too. In the end, Jessica gave blood just fine, though she sobbed the whole time. Lauren left with a few poke marks in her arm, but no blood work. With my luck, she's probably the match, I thought, when they all told me the story later that night.

The next day it was the older cousins' turn. My mom and Meghan drove in from Huntington with a Suburban full—Erik, Mark, and Kristen, my cousins from Massachusetts, their mother, Missy, and my California cousin Jill, who had her two little kids, Sammy and Sarah, with her. I took a peaceful cab ride up from my apartment and met them on the fourth floor. My family is very tall—the average height of our field trip crew was 6 feet (Mark is 6'5")—so we didn't exactly blend in with all the shriveled old people and waifish cancer patients. And between the excitement for the wedding and the anxiety about the blood tests, we weren't too quiet either. Everyone was hoping that they'd be the match. Jill, who's very herby and goddessy, said she had a ghost-like vision come to her and tell her that she was it. But we all knew my only real chance was Meghan. After everyone got their arms wrapped up, we piled back into the Suburban and headed home, ignoring Mark's plea to see Madame Tussaud's wax museum. We had nail appointments and a wedding rehearsal to get to.

Later that night at the rehearsal dinner, I asked my dad if he was nervous for the wedding, to walk down the aisle with Melissa, to give away his first born.

"Since I found out about you, nothing fazes me anymore," he said.

This was a major statement coming from a man who once jumped overboard after a steak he was cooking on his little boat grill fell into the water. He said hearing that I had leukemia was like being hit over the head with a sledgehammer—after that, nothing could feel as bad.

"But I'm not worried about you at all," he quickly added. He was so afraid to let me think he was the slightest bit concerned about my health. He had to act like everything was fine, when clearly it wasn't. Usually my mom was the rock, the one who kept it all together. But now she was stumped. Broken bones, scrapes, fevers, cramps, viruses, sunburns. Those she was good at. Those she could handle. But cancer was going to require more than a warm bath and Saltines; she hated that she couldn't make it all better. And I didn't make it any easier on her, either. If I was heading to Sloan for an appointment and I couldn't find a cab, I'd call my mom in tears, wondering how life could be so cruel. "Couldn't someone stop for me? I'm just trying to get to the hospital. I have cancer," I'd sob into my cell phone from the middle of Times Square. She'd try to calm me down, but what could she say? Eventually my dad asked me to stop calling her when I was so upset. He said she was crying herself to sleep every night. He told me to call him instead, to tell him about not being able to find a cab, or not having anything to wear, but not my mom. She'd had enough.

I was the first one to walk down the aisle, which made me

a bit nervous since the bridesmaid's dresses were so freakin' long. When I was practicing my walk in the back of the church, my heel kept catching the dress and all I could picture was me tripping and the whole church panicking that I'd had a cancer fit. They'd all leap up from their pews and come running to the rescue. I was praying that I wouldn't fall, but the aisle was so long and my feet were numb from being forced to stand outside to take a billion pictures. Despite the 30-degree weather, I wasn't going to wear panty hose with open-toed shoes. I worked at *Glamour* for crying out loud! I'd rather freeze than be a *Glamour* Don't. I bobbled twice but I smiled the whole time, so it was OK.

During the ceremony, I just went through the motions. Sit, stand, kneel, pray. I didn't even cry when Melissa walked down the aisle. I felt completely detached from the whole thing, like Molly Ringwald in *Sixteen Candles.* I even zoned out a few times. Then the intentions of the mass were read. When I heard, "For the sick, especially Erin Zammett, let us pray," I lost it. I couldn't even say the response, "Lord hear our prayer." I just held my breath and let the tears roll down my cheeks until I had to breathe. From behind, I'm sure everyone could tell that I was crying, that my shoulders were shaking in silent sobs. I gasped a little and let out a small cry and then I was able to take deep breaths again and regain my bridesmaid composure. Meghan was crying, too. It was just so strange to hear a packed church praying for me. I appreciated God's help, of course, but it also made me feel like I had no control over the cancer, like I was so screwed that all we could do now is pray for a miracle.

It had been two weeks since I got back from OHSU and still no word on the trials opening. Dr. Cathcart had agreed that the Interferon combination sounded good and she'd be willing to work with Dr. Mauro on the trial so that I wouldn't have to fly to Portland for every finger stick I needed. I was so thankful for her opinion—and her support. I'd been worried she'd be hurt that I went to Oregon, like I was cheating on her. But she was just eager for me to get started. The hydroxyurea had done its job so my blood counts were stable. Because I was in chronic phase I did have some time to play with, but she didn't want me to wait too much longer before beginning the treatment. I didn't want to wait either. The anticipation was awful, like slinking into a cold pool toe by toe, instead of just jumping right in. Sure it was nice to feel so normal that I'd sometimes forget I had anything wrong with me, but the truth was, I'd rather feel a little sick if it meant I'd be getting well.

Up to that point, the hardest part about having cancer was trying to make sense of the fact that I had a big, bad disease coursing through my veins, without so much as a bruise to show for it. (The rash from the hydroxurea had gone away after about a week.) It confused other people, too. A few days before Melissa's wedding, I ran into one of my parents' neighbors at Tortilla Grill. He looked at me all concerned and said, "How is your sister?" I smiled and told him I was the one with leukemia and I was doing great. We all look so much alike so it was an easy mistake to make, but it felt strange, like for a second we were all worried about someone else. It would be just as feasible for Meghan to have leukemia, or Melissa. But I was so glad it wasn't them, or anyone else in my family. So far cancer was easy, but I knew it wouldn't stay that way and I couldn't imagine having to watch someone I love deal with it.

The wedding was a huge success. Melissa and Ysrael looked like movie stars, my parents beamed with pride, and my Uncle B.J., who's about 6'4" and 350 pounds, breakdanced. Everyone had a blast. Ysrael's best man couldn't get a visa to come from Venezuela so Ysrael asked Nick to stand in for him. Nick took the job very seriously and gave a hilarious and touching speech. I was so proud of him and couldn't help thinking that he looked damned good in a tux. I just hoped that we could get through the cancer stuff, because I really wanted to be married to him someday. We had so much fun that night, partying like we didn't have a care in the world. I even had some champagne and danced the salsa with Ysrael (until Melissa cut in). The night couldn't have gone better and it was exactly what we all needed. A nice calm in the storm.

Life (and cancer) go on 4

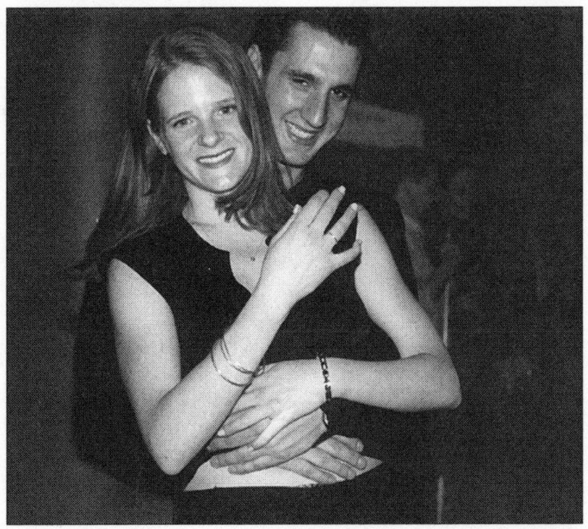

Joking around with my boyfriend, Nick, at my 24th birthday party

WHEN I WAS FIRST DIAGNOSED, I THOUGHT THAT THE only thing that mattered was surviving. But as the weeks ticked by and we were still waiting for the trial to open, I started thinking: There was a possibility that someday this whole cancer thing would be behind me. Or at least on the very back burner. And I knew if that were the case, I would really want to have children. I also knew that my treatment might screw that up for me. I didn't want to be greedy and start thinking about kids before I even took my first dose of Gleevec, but I also didn't want to look back and regret not doing whatever I could to prevent that from happening. Since no one knew for sure how Gleevec affected a woman's fertility, I decided I would have my eggs frozen before I started treatment—get them out and on ice so they couldn't be contaminated. I hadn't spent my whole life doing the right thing just to have the health of my unborn children compromised by some cancer drug. Nick and my parents were far more concerned with *my* health than with the health of my eggs, but they agreed it could be a good preventative measure and that I should start doing some research.

It didn't take much digging to find out that egg freezing was not, in fact, an option. Dr. Cathcart had given me the number of some fancy doctor who specialized in cancer and fertility and he filled me in on a minor little detail. They like to freeze *embryos*, not eggs. (Even in the last three years, the technology of egg freezing has advanced but it still has a low likelihood of success.) This was an interesting twist. You see, an embryo requires sperm, which to me meant that Nick and I would have to decide right then if we were going to get married and have kids together. Though we rarely talked about it, deep down I think we both knew we wanted to marry each other someday. We just didn't want to be one of those couples that picks out their kids' names on their third date and plans their wedding before they've had their first fight. We didn't want to count our chickens before they hatched, so to speak. Sure, it was fun to fantasize about our life together—and sometimes we couldn't help but picture what kind of house we would have or what type of parents we'd be. But talking about our future too much always put a strange pressure on things, like any fight we'd have would be that much more serious because we had already agreed on what color Range Rover we'd drive the kids to soccer practice in. So we tried to avoid it. Plus, we—and by we I mostly mean Nick—had some growing up to do. We were too young, too unsettled in our lives, especially financially. Whenever we were grilled by our family and friends, we'd say, "If we're as in love and as compatible as we are now in three or four years, then we'll do it." We were big on throwing in the "if": *If* we're still together, *if* we still love each other, *if* we get married. But once the embryo stuff came up, we no longer had the luxury of if.

Of course, as the doctor kindly pointed out, I could just

use donor sperm as many women did. That would make Nick feel really good, I thought. It would be like cheating on him, only much more high tech and without the sex. I told the doctor that I had a serious boyfriend and we hoped to get married eventually, we just didn't think we'd be making that decision today. "Uh huh," he said as if he'd heard that a million times. I felt like I needed to defend my relationship, to prove to this guy that Nick and I really were in love and even though we were young, we weren't stupid. We *would* wind up together, he'd see.

The doctor explained that he would likely do an in vitro fertilization, which would require me to give myself hormone injections so I would overproduce eggs. Then he would extract the eggs (not through my belly button as I had originally thought, thank God) and mix them with the sperm to make embryos. Of course it wouldn't be that simple. He wanted me to come in for an actual consultation, so he could run a bunch of tests and give me a clearer picture of what the procedure would entail. He also mentioned that it was an expensive undertaking—$10-12,000 for the one-month cycle of drugs and tests and the procedure and then $1,000 a year to freeze the embryos, which, since I was only 23, would probably wind up being another $10,000. And insurance rarely covered any of it. I was quickly learning that having cancer was not cheap.

When I got off the phone with the fertility guy I called Nick to tell him that they don't freeze eggs, they freeze embryos, and that many women get donor sperm, but that I told the doctor I have a serious boyfriend.

"And, is that a question?" he asked.

"Well, no," I replied, "I'm just telling you what he said. So what do you think?"

"Well there's nothing really to think about. Of course we'll do it," he said.

"I know," I said. But I really wasn't so sure.

I was secretly a little trepidatious about making petri dish babies with a guy I wasn't married to—even if that guy was Nick. I mean what if things started going badly with us? Would I be more inclined to tolerate problems because we'd have the unborn children to think about? If we started fighting about what to get for dinner, would I say, "How can you do this to the embryos?" What if I wound up marrying some other guy and he and I wanted to have children? Would we have to have Nick's kid? All of the mother hens at my office seemed to think that Nick and I should have been having "discussions" about our "feelings" concerning all of this, but what was there to talk about? Nick seemed confident about it and, I finally realized, that was enough for me. Once you have cancer, you just do what you have to do. No matter how weird and costly that might be. My mom told me she'd love to be the first one on the block with a test tube grandkid, and later that night, Nick and I toasted to the embryos. I made the appointment for the following week. At the very least it would be fodder for my *Glamour* story.

Meanwhile, Melissa, who was probably more concerned about the kid thing than the cancer thing, told me that she and Ysrael discussed it and she would be happy to carry my children for me if I couldn't do it myself. Whoa. It sounded a little *Lifetime Movie of the Week* for me. Did I want kids *that* badly? For Melissa, I knew nothing could be worse than not being able to have children—this was a girl who used to breast feed her baby dolls. And all those times that I was playing with my Barbies (and Barbie wasn't getting her hair done), Melissa was off playing house with Meghan. Melissa was always the mom—that was the only way she'd play—and she took her role very seriously, making pretend bottles and changing pretend diapers and burping pretend burps. She couldn't wait to be a real mother. And while part of her concern was definitely rooted in the fact that if I couldn't have kids, her 17 kids would have no cousins to grow up with, it was really nice of her to offer her uterus. I just doubted I would go that far. If I couldn't at least carry my own babies, then I'd adopt. Or have dogs.

A few weeks into the New Year, Dr. Mauro called with news: "An issue has arisen that may preclude you from participating in the Interferon trial," he said in his best doctorspeak. Though all my blood tests had checked out, he was concerned with my medical history, specifically my ITP history. Apparently Interferon can aggravate autoimmune diseases and since I'd had one—even though it was 15 years ago—there was a chance I could develop it again. If the ITP did come back, I'd have to stop the CML treatment and treat the ITP, which would be at best a huge pain in the ass (my words, not Dr. Mauro's) and at worst, undermine the success of my treatment (his words). He said that he and Dr. Druker were going to discuss it further and he'd keep me posted. He could tell by the tone of my voice that I felt defeated. "We'll know something soon," he said. The Ara-C trial was still a good option to consider and that one was supposed to open up any day now. He'd call me as soon as he knew anything. Soon, he said. Again.

With the holidays over, everything at work was pretty much back to normal. Most of my coworkers knew about my CML and would check up on me periodically. I completely appreciated their concern, but sometimes it was tough to tell if a "how are you?" was just a "how are you?" or if it was a "how *are* you?" The one time I misjudged that question it led to a 30-minute conversation with one of our reporters in the elevator bank. Apparently she was just making polite conversation. I thought she wanted a cancer update. She was shocked, of course, when I answered her question by saying that my blood counts had stabilized but I was still waiting for the clinical trial in Oregon to open up. Say what? Then I had to stand there and explain everything from the beginning which took a while since I was incapable of telling the story without also mentioning what I was wearing the day I was diagnosed (dressy tan pants and a tan shirt from Zara) and what I ate for dinner after I found out (loaded nachos). It didn't bother me, of course. My cancer was constantly on my mind, and I figured the more people who knew, the easier it would be on me—and them. A few weeks after I was diagnosed, a friend had sent balloons and a little get-well bear to the office. I had them sitting on my desk, and random people kept walking by saying, "Oh, is it your birthday?" I really didn't want to have to say to some poor fashion department intern, "No, it's not my birthday. I have leukemia," but I didn't want to lie either. In a way I wished my editor-in-chief had sent a company-wide e-mail: "Just wanted to let everyone know that Erin Zammett, the redhead who sits in the pod, has leukemia now. OK, back to work." Unless I told people, they'd have no idea there was anything wrong with me. And even when they did know, it was hard to believe. When I first came back from Christmas vacation, one rather frank editor said, "Oh my God, you look great! I was expecting you to look all sickly and pale and cancer-like." Yeah, you and me both.

For the most part, I still felt as good as I looked. There was only one day that I wasn't really 100 percent but I couldn't figure out if it was because of the CML or if it was just a cold. I supposed having cancer didn't disqualify me from catching whatever it was that had everyone else at the office popping cough drops and running to the drug store for Puffs Plus, but it was hard to imagine that cancer didn't have something to do with my being under the weather. I mean once you have cancer, is a headache ever really just a headache anymore? I was tired and achy, like someone had taken a baseball bat to my body. If I didn't already know that I had cancer, I would have said something dramatic like, "I think I'm dying." Normally when I felt that way, I'd try to push through it, put on a cute outfit and suck it up. Instead, I spent the entire day lying on my bed watching *The Real World Hawaii*—the first 14 episodes. Doing nothing was a new experience for me and I can't say I hated it. I did, however, hate Amaya. God was she a pain in the ass. And as I laid there eating an ice cream sandwich and marveling at just how drunk Ruthie could get, I wondered if MTV would want me to be on *The Real World.* The true story of a real life cancer patient. It would be good drama. I could be like Pedro, except hopefully I would live in the end.

The appointment with the fertility specialist turned out to be a $400 flop. From the moment I walked into his office, I felt uncomfortable, like I didn't belong. The other women in the waiting room were there with husbands, or at the very least, wedding bands, and they looked all serious and maternal. I was there with my mom, my *US Weekly* and my Diet Coke. And I immediately disliked the doctor. First, he was a little tactless: "Whose property will the embryos be if you don't survive the cancer?" he actually asked within the first five minutes of our sitting down in his office. Hmm. Hadn't really thought of that one yet. It was a valid question, though. What if something did happen to me? Would the embryos go to Nick or my parents? The whole thing felt weird and I started to wonder why I was even there. Then he brought up the ethical issues, like what to do with any embryos I didn't use. Being Catholic I was probably supposed to say I would put up the embryos for adoption or something, but frankly, I didn't have time for ethics. Since I had gotten cancer everything became medical to me, so I told the doctor that if I couldn't use them, they could just be destroyed.

The kicker was that after the doctor ran some tests—external *and* internal—and told us that everything looked fine, he said he highly doubted I'd be able to do the in vitro. The problem was, before I could harvest my eggs I'd have to flush the hydroxurea completely out of my system, which would mean going off the drug for at least two menstrual cycles. And I just couldn't do that. Despite how good I felt, I had cancer and without the hydroxurea keeping my counts in check, that cancer would make me very sick. In other words, going to see this guy was a big, fat waste of time. The thing that pissed me off the most was that I'd told the doctor I was on hydroxyurea when I spoke with him on the phone. Why couldn't he have saved us the trip and the disappointment? And the $400—which, as predicted, was not covered by my insurance. Before we left he told us about some creepy experimental procedure he was working on which, if I remember correctly, involved removing an ovary, freezing it, then slicing it up and putting it back in the patient's arm. I told him thanks but no thanks. We were done.

When I told Nick the news all he said was, "I'd rather not have kids than not have you." Hearing him say that made me cry. Since I had been diagnosed I felt a little like damaged goods, and after failing at the embryo thing, I *really* did. But to Nick, I was still a catch. He had told me many times before that I was the most important thing in his life, but I also knew he really wanted to be a dad. I was telling him that might never happen and he was completely unfazed by it. "All I care about is you getting better," he said. As much I loved him for saying that, I hated to think that I, that *we*, might not be able to experience everything life had to offer.

I felt the need to buy something expensive to cheer myself up. Since being diagnosed, I had become quite the shopper. If I can't have kids then I should at least have Prada shoes, I thought. Despite the fact that I lived in Manhattan and worked at a fashion magazine, and was a woman, I had never really loved shopping. I only went to the mall when I needed something and even then, I was practical, always checking out the sale racks first, avoiding Saks and Bergdorf like the plague. Then I got cancer. Suddenly I felt the urge to accessorize. Expensively. I had to have a $300 Coach bag. And a Tiffany ring. And Donna Karan sunglasses. Of course I wasn't making a salary that could pay for such luxuries, but I adopted my mother's new favorite saying and spoiled myself a little (and, OK, if my mom offered, which she often did those days, I'd let her pick up the tab). While I knew that retail therapy wasn't going to cure my cancer, looking at my fabulous new stuff did make me feel really good. And that had to mean something.

I also found myself tipping cab drivers and waitresses more, adding an extra dollar here and there. What the hell, I thought, it's only money. Plus, I wanted people to think kindly of me, to send nice thoughts about me into the universe. After my blow-up with Meghan, I figured I could use all the good karma I could get. I was constantly asking Nick if he thought I was a good person before all this happened, if he thought I was decent. In some ways I felt like I was running for office, like I needed everyone to like me so I could get their vote. Then I could take a petition to the cancer gods and say, "C'mon guys, look how many people want me to get better" and they'd say, "Ah, yes, quite an impressive list you've got here. No more cancer for you." Really, I just wanted to know that I had people on my side and that they would root for me, that even though a very bad thing had happened, good things were still possible.

They were. At a mid-January appointment with Dr. Cathcart, we found out that Meghan was my perfect bone marrow match. Except for hearing that my cancer was gone, that was the best news I could have asked for. My mom started crying as Dr. Cathcart read us the details of the results. Meghan was an identical six for six HLA match. There was nothing better. I just said, "That's great," and then told them about the dream I'd had the night before. In my dream, I'd asked Dr. Cathcart's assistant to look up the bone marrow results for me. She wasn't supposed to, but she did it anyway and found out that Meghan was a 110 percent match. I remembered feeling so excited but also so scared that Dr. Cathcart would get mad at me for breaking the rules. I was psychic! Sort of, anyway. Dr. Cathcart said she didn't think it was possible to be a 110 percent match and we all laughed. Then we discussed the new options this development introduced.

Though we had all already agreed that I would do the Interferon trial (or the Ara-C trial if the Interferon people banned me), Dr. Cathcart thought it would be a good idea for me to meet with a transplant doctor so I would be fully aware of all of my options. She set up an appointment for a few days later. She's good like that, always laying it all out on the table, always looking out for my best interests. She also said if the trial in Oregon didn't open up soon, we had to go to plan B, Gleevec alone. "It's time to fish or cut bait," she said. There was a chance the disease could be progressing, and I'd need more specific treatment soon. In the meantime, my mom and I went to the diner across the street for chocolate chip pancakes to celebrate Meghan's matching marrow.

"I knew it!" Meghan said when I called her between mouthfuls with the news. She told me that she'd had a feeling, but didn't want to curse it so she'd never mentioned it. Then she asked me what being my match meant for her. "Can I still drink?" she asked. There was actually nothing she could—or couldn't—do that would affect her bone marrow, but I let her believe that she needed to start taking better care of herself. For years I had been trying to get her to live a healthier life—I don't think she had broken a sweat since she quit soccer when she was eight years old—and I figured this might be just the incentive she needed to make a change. She was drinking too much and smoking too much and eating too much and not exercising at all. Meghan and I couldn't be more different, which made it really hard to believe that our marrow was essentially the same. But I didn't question it. I just hoped that if I ever did need the transplant I wouldn't get any of her lazy cells.

The marrow news came at a good time for Meghan. She had just failed Spanish and though her bad grades were no longer the family crisis they once were (cancer will do that), she was still getting the "what the hell happened?" lectures. But now she was the hero. She could have dropped out of school that week and it wouldn't have mattered. Of course, of all the subjects to fail, Spanish was not ideal. She had been begging my parents to send her to Spain to take advanced language classes for the summer and until her grades came out, they had been on the fence about letting her go. The F pushed them right to the "what are you, nuts? You're not going anywhere" side of the fence. Though I couldn't quite comprehend how she could fail *any* class, let alone Spanish, I did feel bad for her. Meghan had the uncanny ability to get sympathy in any situation. She was the martyr in the family. No matter how at fault she was, she always came off as the victim. She'd just look at you with her giant doe eyes, like she was clueless, maybe even whip up some dramatic tears, and you couldn't help but feel like she was the sweetest, most misunderstood person around. Still, I was glad she wasn't going to party it up in Madrid for the summer. I wanted her bone marrow close to home.

That afternoon, Meghan actually went running and did Tae Bo. "It's weird, I'm living for two now," she said when she called to tell me about her workout. In a strange way, she was right. If anything happened to Meghan, I would not only be affected emotionally, but physically, too. I told her not to fall off any cliffs. Fortunately, she had just quit her flying lessons. She had been training to be a pilot, but it turned out to be yet another of her short-lived career goals. She changed her mind a few months into the lessons, despite the fact that my father had spent thousands on state-of-the-art flight equipment. He hadn't learned his lesson when the darkroom he set up for her in high school got used three times before becoming a full-time dust collector. Meghan was a good kid, but she had no idea what she wanted to do with her life, so whenever she showed interest in anything, my parents got excited and overindulged her "passion." It was easy to see how they got duped. When she was into something, Meghan became like a used car salesman. She had extremely convincing pitches for how she was going to be a veterinarian, a wedding planner, a pharmacist, a makeup artist. But the truth was, the only activity Meghan took any real and consistent interest in was shopping.

Growing up, my family would spend every February break in Boca Raton with Grandma Ruth, my dad's mom. That's where Meghan first learned to shop. On the days when Melissa and I would go golfing with my dad, my grandma, whose two favorite things were spending money and spoiling her grandkids, would take Meghan to the Town Center, the biggest, most beautiful mall any of us had ever seen (my mom would go to the pool for a few hours of cherished alone time). It wasn't unheard of for them to come home with a trunk-full of shopping bags. They got clothes, purses, jewelry, *everything*. On one particularly successful trip, Grandma Ruth bought Meghan 13 pairs of shoes, which they had spread out in the living room for all of us to see. When we got home from the golf course, my father nearly tripped over the jelly shoes and patent leathers and multi-colored Keds that stretched across the floor—and he almost blew his top when he realized the extent of their little spree. Then Grandma Ruth and Meghan looked at each other, giggled and confessed that there had been a two-for-one sale at KMart and they got the whole lot for under $50. My grandma, who usually filled our Florida closets with Polly Flinders and Lilly Pulitzer and Laura Ashley, couldn't resist a blue light special. Melissa and I were always a little jealous of Meghan's loot, of course, but then we'd just tell her how Daddy let us drive the golf cart when the ranger wasn't looking. And bought us lemonades and frozen Snickers bars from the clubhouse. And let us steer the rental car on the way home. So there.

When I called Dr. Mauro with the bone marrow news he was thrilled: "The world is your oyster," he said. I had always believed that the world was my oyster, but he meant my oyster in terms of cancer treatment, which wasn't quite the same thing. He had good news too: He and Dr. Druker had decided that I could do the Interferon trial after all; the risk of the ITP coming back was negligible. I later realized that Dr. Mauro tended to be a little conservative, which is why he brought up the ITP issue in the first place. Neither Dr. Druker nor Dr. Cathcart had been concerned about it at all. But my being let back in didn't matter anyway since the trial still hadn't started. I told Dr. Mauro about the fishing or cutting bait thing and he agreed. It was time to make a move. We talked for a while about all of my options and finally decided to just pick a date and book my trip to Oregon. If the Interferon trial wasn't open by the time I got out there, I'd start the Ara-C trial, which had just opened and had already enrolled several patients. Though I had felt strongly about doing the Interferon trial at first, there was really little scientific difference behind the two combinations. And at that point, I didn't really care. I just wanted to do something other than hydroxurea—ever since Dr. Cathcart told me it was like a Band-Aid, I couldn't help thinking it was a bit useless, like we were treating a severed limb with a tiny piece of Johnson&Johnson plastic.

With a date in the calendar, everything became very real very quickly. On February 14—Valentine's Day—my mom and I would fly to Portland. There would be tests and monitoring and tutorials before I could officially start the trial, so we'd be staying out there for almost two weeks. Wanting to prepare myself as much as possible for the impending suckiness, I called Dr. Mauro to ask him about all the side effects of the Gleevec, the one drug I knew I'd be taking. Despite the media's portrayal, this little orange pill wasn't quite as gentle as a vitamin. There were many potential reactions, but they all depended on the person, the dose, the drug combination, the severity of the disease, etc. I might experience all of them and I might not experience any. Dr. Mauro told me that in the beginning, I could definitely expect some muscle cramping and bone pain, but it would go away, he said. I was fine with that. And I was OK with the possible indigestion and the nausea too. In fact the only side effect that really haunted me was the water retention or "puffiness." Dr. Mauro sort of implied that being young and working at *Glamour*, I may care about my appearance more than some of his other patients, who, for the most part, were older men and women (and pretty much guaranteed not to work in the Condé Nast building). "You might look like you haven't slept in a few days," he said about the potential swelling around the eyes and lips. "And there may be swelling around the ankles, too." Lovely. Dr. Mauro said we could control the swelling with diuretics, but I wasn't comforted. If you have to have cancer, you should at least be able to look skinny. Talk about adding insult to injury. Dr. Mauro told me not to worry. He'd see me in a few weeks.

Meanwhile, I had some partying to do. January 30th was my 24th birthday and I had planned a huge bash to celebrate. My so-called normal life was literally going on, and I figured a party would be the perfect way to show everyone that I was still me, that despite what that bitch from high school said, I was not dying, I was living—and drinking beer to boot! It would also be a last hurrah before heading to Portland to start treatment (and before turning into Puffy McGee). The party was planned for the Saturday after my birthday at a cool new billiards lounge in my neighborhood and everyone was invited. My college friend Amy was even coming up from Nashville to help me hostess. There'd be a *Glamour* photographer there, of course, which meant that I had to find the perfect outfit. And get my hair cut. And get my nails done. I was so excited.

On my actual birthday, a Wednesday, Nick took me out for a low-key dinner at Mesa Grill, the Southwestern restaurant owned by Bobby Flay from the Food Network. We talked about how much we would miss each other and how lucky we were to have each other and how I would bring him back an Oregon Ducks hat. Then we had our usual conversation about how surreal the whole cancer thing was.

"I still can't believe you have cancer," he said. "It just sucks."

"I know," I said. "Can you imagine if I *died*? That would *really* suck." I meant it as a joke, albeit a sick, morbid cancer joke, but it didn't go over so well.

"Jesus, Erin."

"I'm just saying . . . I think if I am going to die we should get engaged so that you get proper sympathy ya know? Otherwise no one will realize how serious we were."

"I know, right. I'd just be the random boyfriend. "

"Anyway, I'm not going to die so it doesn't really matter."

"Good, I'm glad."

"Thanks."

The actor Phillip Seymour Hoffman was sitting at a table near ours, which was cool, but other than that it was a quiet night. We were saving our energy for the weekend and we had done the family cake thing a few days earlier when we were out on Long Island for my Grandma Del's birthday party. She and I have the same birthday, and she turned 80 that year, so all of my aunts and uncles came in to town to celebrate with her. My parents threw a really nice dinner in her honor, and everyone had a good time. But we weren't allowed to call too much attention to the number of candles on the cake. Grandma Del didn't believe in birthdays. If you asked her age (which my sisters and I often did, just to get a rise out of her) she'd shush you or tell you she was 29 again. And some days I think she believed it. Even at 80 she was in amazing shape—she danced, golfed, swam and did sit-ups and leg lifts every single day. She also cooked and cleaned for my grandfather who was just about the coolest guy around, but totally clueless when it came to domestic duties. She was a Radio City Rockette in the 1940s and still kicked like one. She had run a dancing school out of her house for 30 years (Meghan, Melissa and I all took lessons); she'd only given it up a year earlier. *Glamour* had just featured her in a cute story called "Sex Advice from Women Who Have Been Doing it for

Decades" or something like that. Of course Grandma Del said that she didn't even know what "the sex act" was when she came to New York City and all the advice she gave was prefaced with "kids these days . . . ," but she loved being in the magazine. And she looked awesome. Because of her showbiz background she was very aware of her looks and absolutely hated getting old. In fact, that was all she talked about that night. Wrinkles, wrinkles and more wrinkles.

The next day, though, she had a change of heart. "I should be proud of my age," she told me when she called to thank my mom for the party. "I should have said that I hope all of my children and grandchildren live as long as I have." I think she felt bad because she realized that she was turning 80 and was still in perfect health, while I was only turning 24 and already had leukemia. She was lucky and she knew it. I would give anything to live a long, healthy life and still be kicking at 80. Grandma Del had always been my role model and I told her that. I also told her that if I ever did have kids, I would give one of them the middle name Adele. She still hadn't gotten over the fact that after being born on her birthday, I wasn't named after her. I actually think Erin Adele would have been pretty, but I'm Erin Elizabeth. Oh well. I did give one of my Cabbage Patch kids the name Adele Ruth, after my two grandmas, but I suppose that didn't count.

My birthday party in the city was awesome. Everyone showed up—work friends, city friends, Long Island friends—and partied well into the night. Even me. I think some of my less-enlightened guy friends from high school had a tough time seeing me have so much fun, dancing and laughing and shooting pool like a normal person. Didn't I have cancer? Shouldn't I be home in bed? It was also hard for them to talk to me about the cancer, for them to accept that this was happening to someone like me. I was prom queen for crying out loud! If "Least Likely To Get Cancer" had been a category in our senior yearbook, I would have been named it.

My teetotaling days had ended about a month into my diagnosis, but I was still drinking only beer. Somehow slugging dirty martinis, my pre-CML favorite, didn't quite go with the whole cancer persona, so I adopted beer as my new drink of choice. It seemed like the healthiest option—wasn't it made from potatoes or something? Of course I had about six Sierra Nevadas that night, which I realized was not healthy and certainly not what my doctors meant by moderation. But after spending most of my life drinking shitty light beer, I hadn't realized how good a good beer could actually be. I was feeling very cancer free and I lost track. Naturally I regretted it the next morning and proceeded to beat myself up a little. I mean, what kind of cancer patient has a hangover? I felt like a loser. A cancer loser. But, whatever, I'd had fun. And who knew when the next time I could do that would be.

A few days after my birthday, I got a long-awaited promotion—from editorial assistant to assistant editor. My title didn't sound much different, and I'd still be answering Alison's phone, but the change was a big deal to me. Most importantly it meant that I finally had business cards to give out at all the book lunches and parties I went to (the old "Oh, I don't have any cards with me today" routine was getting old). But being promoted so soon after my diagnosis was a little weird—I worried people would think it was a pity promotion, like Cindi was throwing me a bone to make up for the fact that I had a potentially deadly disease. She wasn't, of course, not at all. I worked hard for *Glamour* and completely deserved to move up the masthead, but I couldn't help feeling a little strange. Promotions were hard to come by and magazine people have a way of making you feel like you should actually be paying *them* to work there. So when you do get a promotion, you almost feel guilty, like you should say, "Oh, thanks, but no thanks. I really don't deserve this. Why don't you keep it for yourself?" It sounds crazy, I know, but that's the business. And every penny that you make (and it is pennies) is considered a gift, and you should be thankful, grateful, even, despite the fact that you're at work till 10 p.m., you don't make overtime and it's never enough to pay the rent.

I think part of the reason I felt so weird about the promotion was because I was leaving for Oregon a few days later. Of course I had a really good reason to be out of the office for two weeks (hel-lo, cancer!), and the magazine could certainly run without me—and, I should add, no one was giving me a hard time about going—but the timing just sucked. Still, I was excited about my new title and put a rush order on my business cards so I could bring them with me to Oregon. You never know who you're going to meet at a cancer hospital. Plus, I wanted to show them to my mom.

The day before I left for Portland, Alison took me to lunch. We talked about my promotion and my journal writing and my expectations about the trial. As she paid the check, she said, "So, am I being OK about everything? Am I asking the right questions and talking about the cancer enough but not too much? That sort of thing?" It was so nice of her to ask, but I didn't really know what to say. I thought she was being fine to me, but how the hell would I know? I was no expert on cancer talk. There are no behavioral guidelines that come with your diagnosis, no *Glamour* Dos & Don'ts. I didn't even know if *I* was acting appropriately. If I had to guess, I'd say I was a little too flip about the whole thing, guzzling too many beers, telling too many jokes, talking about it too candidly (case in point: the scene at the elevator). I'm sure my attitude made people uncomfortable sometimes, but the truth was, I didn't know how else to be.

Though we all knew I wouldn't be opting for a transplant, my parents and I went to the meeting Dr. Cathcart had set up with an open mind. The transplant doctor, another young, pretty woman, took us through the entire procedure, painful step by painful step. When you have a transplant, you're essentially getting a whole new immune system—in my case, I'd be getting Meghan's—and in order to prepare your body to accept it, they have to first kill off your entire existing immune system. They do this with heavy chemotherapy and radiation. Conditioning, it's called. And during it you're highly susceptible to infection—a normally harmless bacteria could kill you. Once you've survived that, they give you the donor marrow, which is not actually planted into your body in some high-tech, sci-fi way, but given to you in a drip from an IV. "It's surprisingly anticlimactic," the doctor said, trying to be funny, I think. Then you wait and see if the donor marrow takes and starts building the new immune system you so desperately need at that point.

The procedure requires an average of about four to six weeks in the hospital. Then, for a whole year, you're under intense medical scrutiny. And you can't be around crowds unless you wear a mask and you're constantly treating the many lovely symptoms of "graft versus host disease," which is a very common side effect that occurs when the patient's body fights the donor marrow. Sweet, I thought, and stopped listening. I just couldn't hear any more. What if I had to do this some day? Did I really want to know about all the awful things that could happen to me? Instead, I focused on the golf-ball sized diamond ring on the doctor's finger and thought about Billy Crudup, who I'd seen at the bagel store down the street from Sloan before the meeting. He was very cute, but like most Hollywood heartthrobs, much shorter than you'd think.

In the end, the doctor said it was worth starting treatment with Gleevec. She told us that it was best to do a transplant within 18 months of diagnosis, so I could join the trial and if after six months or so, the results weren't great, I'd still be within that window. God, I hoped the Gleevec would work.

The night before I left, Nick came into the city and we went to Blue Water Grill for a pre-Valentine's Day dinner. We never used to go to so many nice restaurants, but since I'd been diagnosed, we figured what the hell, it's only money. He bought me a dozen red roses, which was a nice gesture, but a little silly considering I was getting on an airplane the next day. I had to bite my tongue not to tell him he'd wasted his money. God, I was hard to please. He also made me a mix CD for the trip, which he reluctantly let me preview later that night while I finished packing. All of the songs were great, but they were all sort of sad. Or maybe we were just sad. Everything had been so good between us lately and we knew that was about to change. When I got back from Portland, I'd be on Gleevec, no turning back.

The line "How wonderful life is while you're in the world" from Elton John's "Your Song" blared out of my stereo and I started crying. It brought up the idea of not being in the world and that sucked. I asked Nick if he'd seriously thought about that possibility at all and he said in the beginning, me dying was all he could think about. He said he used to lie awake at night picturing himself standing next to my parents at my grave with dark sunglasses on. Jesus, I had no idea. Suddenly I felt really bad for ever joking about it with him. But I guess I couldn't blame him for being so morbid. I mean I did have cancer and despite the fact that I'd been chugging beers a few days earlier, it was pretty serious. But I just wouldn't let my mind go there. I never could.

When I was in seventh grade, my English teacher, Mr. McKay, gave the class an assignment to write our own obituary. I told him I thought that was cruel and got a pass to go to the library for the period. But I still lay awake that night thinking about what it meant to die. Ditto when we studied Edgar Allan Poe. And when I accidentally saw *My Girl*, the seemingly kid-friendly movie where Macaulay Culkin dies from bee stings, I didn't think I would recover. I started imagining everyone I loved dying and leaving me behind to throw myself on their coffins like the little girl in the movie did. It was so awful. But as much as I freaked myself out with the idea of death, I never really thought about me being the one to die. Even now that I had cancer.

In fact for the first time since I'd been diagnosed, I started thinking about what it would be like to *not* have leukemia anymore, to be a survivor. I couldn't really picture it, but I knew it would be great to be cancer free. And if Nick and I couldn't have kids, so what, we'd have each other. And our green Range Rover. Of course I had a long road ahead of me, and there were a lot of unknowns, but as my mom and I boarded the plane to Oregon the next afternoon—Nick's roses in hand—I was hopeful. It was the only way to be.

It's official 5

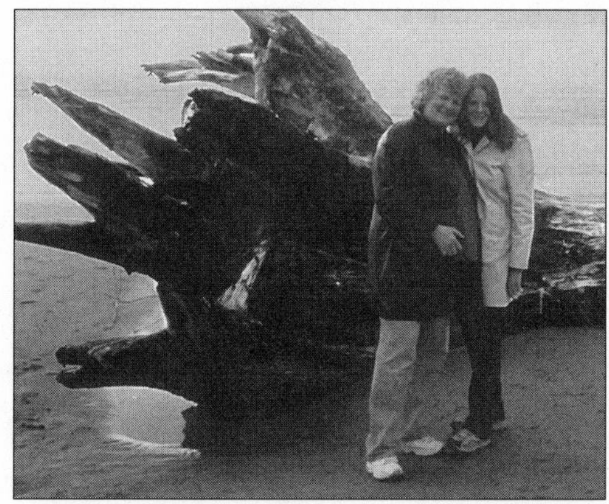

My mom and me (and a big tree) on the beach in Oregon

FEBRUARY IS HANDS-DOWN THE MOST DEPRESSING TIME of year to be in Portland. The sun is nowhere to be seen, the sky is a muddy gray and it is always, always raining. And it's not a stormy, dramatic, driving rain that starts and stops, offering a few hopeful reprieves. It's a constant, light rain, a ubiquitous mist that's there when you wake up and there when you go to bed. I had packed clothes for every possible forecast and every possible occasion but ended up spending most of my time there in a green waterproof Gap pullover I had gotten back in high school. But it wasn't so much the rain that got to me—it was my mother's *reaction* to the rain. Even though everyone told us to expect it, and every night we watched the weatherman call for it, she woke up each morning, walked to the hotel room window, pulled back the curtains and exclaimed, totally defeated, "It's raining again." For some reason this really pissed me off. "Mom, it's going to rain the entire time we're here, that's what it does in Portland, can you please stop acting so surprised by that?" When she'd talk to my dad or my sisters, or email her friends from my laptop (another thing that pissed me off since I had to re-explain how to do it each time), she'd always mention the rain first. In fact, "Still raining" was usually her subject line. Nick had made me promise I'd be nice to her while we were away, and I was trying, but two weeks together in the rain was a lot to ask for.

In typical Type-A fashion I was multitasking the whole time we were out there. Cindi, *Glamour*'s editor-in-chief, had decided she wanted to debut my cancer column as a feature in the May issue (and then run a follow-up every other month after that). It was only February, but in the magazine world that meant that my first draft was due to my editor, Jill, five days after I arrived in Oregon. I planted myself at the desk in our hotel room and tirelessly transcribed my journal, figuring out which details were important to include and which could be cut (sadly, I couldn't turn in 200 pages). Being objective about my story wasn't easy—nor was reliving the diagnosis. It had only been three months, but it already felt like a lifetime. And in some ways, I was over it. I had fully accepted having cancer as a fact of my life, become numb to it even. But reading my journal made it all real again.

It was so painful to remember what it felt like to hear Dr. Lutsky's voice on my answering machine that day and, worse, what it was like to sit in his office and hear him say, "Yes, like leukemia." I cried as I revisited the pay-phone conversation with my mom and the first day at Sloan. Most of the time I wrote through tears. My mom, who was never far away, lying on the bed reading her book or sitting in the chair crocheting a blanket for one of the new babies in our extended family, would catch a glimpse of my red eyes and start crying herself, which would make me even more sad. We had both adopted a "shit happens, we deal with it" attitude, so to see her cry now was like re-opening an old wound. A big one. OK, so I guess it wasn't just the weather that was depressing.

Our first appointment at OHSU was the morning after we flew out and it was just for tests. The interferon trial still wasn't open—surprise, surprise—so I would be joining the Gleevec/ Ara-C trial, but not until they made sure everything from my liver to my bladder was functioning properly. We had John, the *Glamour* photographer who'd been there on our first trip, with us again, which made our visit both more awkward and more bearable. He and his assistant followed me into each little lab, snapping away as the nurse filled huge vials with my blood and plugged me into a heart rate monitor and took my temperature and measured my height and weight. I told him not to shoot the number on the scale, please. Millions of *Glamour* readers didn't need to know how much I weighed. *I* didn't even want to know. But since I'd been diagnosed, I couldn't help it. I'd been weighed about 58 times. I had cancer, not an eating disorder, yet when I'd go to see either of my doctors, the first thing the nurse would do is put me on the scale.

I had lost about eight pounds the first month I was diagnosed—in fact, on that first visit, I told John to shoot the number on the scale, please, because it was the lowest weight I'd been in as long as I could remember. I had been eating much more fattening foods in those first few weeks and exercising a lot less, but somehow, the weight just fell off me. I suppose it was the CML, or the stress caused by the diagnosis, and I shouldn't have been quite so thrilled by it, but I couldn't help it. I thought I looked great (and looking back at pictures from that time, I really did). Now, though, I was right back to where I was the day I went into Dr. Lutsky's office. Damn. Even though technically I hadn't gained eight pounds, I'd just gotten back to my normal weight, I felt like a fat ass. A fat ass with cancer—not a good combination. Though I had always placed more emphasis on my weight than I probably should have—and I was perpetually saying that I needed to lose five pounds—I had given up getting on scales years earlier. I was pretty happy with my body (if a little crazy about it), but I just knew that if I started putting a number on it, I'd become obsessed. And I was right. Now, thanks to my little cancer weigh-ins, I had a potential deadly disease to contend with and a weight complex to boot. As I would go in for checkups over the following year, sometimes I'd find myself more anxious about the number of pounds I weighed than the number of leukemia cells swimming through my body. Sick, I know.

Of course, no day of CML testing would be complete without having the granddaddy of all tests: the bone marrow biopsy. Though you can get a pretty good indication of how the disease is progressing from looking at blood tests, the only way to know for sure is to look directly at the marrow. Doing the biopsy right before I started treatment was a way for Dr. Mauro to establish a baseline to see exactly how much leukemia he was dealing with. Then I'd have a biopsy every three months after that so he could track the disease as the trial progressed. When I first heard about how many biopsies I would be having, I wanted to skip the trial, just take Gleevec and stick with Dr. Cathcart (who'd only be giving a biopsy every six months), but then I found something online that gave me hope. Before the trip, I had Googled Dr. Mauro and a patient-run CML website popped up. It had a page of testimonials on the best doctors and facilities and Dr. Mauro was one of the first people listed. Under his photo was the tagline, "Painless bone marrows!" Yeah, right, I thought at first. At that point I could still feel my insides being pulled out from the biopsy I'd had at Sloan. But as the memory of gripping onto the table for dear life became more and more distant, I started rationalizing. Maybe Dr. Mauro had a different technique. Maybe he used different needles. Maybe I'd even fall asleep on the table. If it was on the Internet it's gotta be true, right?

After explaining how the lab would take tiny amounts of my bone marrow and look at it under a microscope to observe any mutations, Dr. Mauro asked if we had any questions. I had one: "Can we just do the biopsy and then ask questions?" I asked. I had been trying to psych myself up for it, but deep down I was still scared and the anticipation was making it worse. "Not a problem," Dr. Mauro said. Then he asked if I minded having an audience. There were two bigwigs from a drug company observing the hospital that day and Dr. Mauro really wanted them to watch a procedure being done. "What the hell, right?" I said. "The more the merrier." I really didn't care who watched, as long as my mom wasn't in the room. I just didn't want her to see me go through that pain. Plus, if my mommy was with me, I might break down. Or worse, *she* might break down.

She seemed a little disappointed that I didn't want her with me but just shrugged and said she'd get another chapter read. I felt bad, but I really didn't want to make a big deal out of it. I wanted to duck in like I had done at Sloan. Everyone thought I was crazy. If I had drug company strangers and a freakin' camera crew in there, why not the woman who birthed me? "Erin, what's the big deal?" said John, who was a super sweet guy and could just as easily have passed for a Sunday school teacher. "It's your mom, you have to let her in." Even though I knew he had an ulterior motive—pleasing Donald with emotional mother/daughter shots on the biopsy table—he was right. Finally, I relented and told her she could come as long as she promised not to talk about the weather—or tell anyone my life story (my mother would chat up the president if he walked by). She promised to be on her best behavior and when I saw how happy she was to be included, I immediately felt guilty for ever saying I didn't want her in there with me. What kind of daughter was I?

The biopsy was painless as advertised. Of course it may have been that I was expecting such a horrible experience that anything less than a sledgehammer to the head would seem like a tickle, but really, other than having my butt crack on display, I was totally comfortable. Pain, of course, is relative. I felt a few "bee stings" in the beginning when he numbed the area, and a strange pressure, the notion of pain, while he pushed through the bone, but nothing worth gripping the table for. The hardest part was watching my mother, who cringed every time Dr. Mauro cranked, and having Dr. Mauro keep asking me if I felt anything. "OK, you might feel a sharpness in a second," he'd say. I didn't, but knowing that it should hurt freaked me out. That and the fact that my mom would say, "Really? You didn't feel that? Gheesh!"

John had strategically placed my mom right next to my head and at one point he had her put her hand on my face like she was comforting me. That was exactly what I didn't want, but I supposed if we were just faking it for the camera, it was OK. As she started to pet my head, I giggled. The she giggled. Then I giggled more. Then Dr. Mauro said very patiently, like a dentist talking to a five-year-old, "OK, I just need you to be still for another minute here." I loved it. I was actually being reprimanded for being rowdy during my biopsy. I should put that on the website! A few minutes later, Dr. Mauro said, "OK, now just lie there for a little while before you get up." I couldn't believe it. It was over and I was still smiling. Dr. Mauro was smiling too. If bone marrow biopsies were a sport, he would have pumped his fist and high-fived the technician. He'd done a great job and he was proud of himself. "See," he said. "Told ya you'd be fine."

After hands were washed and bandages put in place, we finally got to talk about the trial. The nurse came in with lots of pamphlets and paperwork and walked us through the whole process, step by step. There would be homework, so I had to pay attention. First, the drugs: I would be taking 400 mg (four pills) of Gleevec every single day. She suggested I take them in the morning with my breakfast and plenty of water—the Gleevec tended to make patients a bit nauseated, so I might have to eat more than a piece of toast or a bowl of cereal.

Breakfast was my favorite meal of the day, so I figured I could handle that. Plus, I had the Condé Nast cafeteria at my disposal. I could get a smoked salmon and cream cheese omelet with a side of turkey bacon and a mango smoothie made to order if I needed to. I had the weigh-ins to think about, though, so I'd probably stick with my usual bowl of half oatmeal, half cream of wheat and maybe add a hard-boiled egg or two.

I would take the Gleevec alone for two weeks, then add the shots of Ara-C for two weeks, then Gleevec alone for two weeks and so on and so on. During my two-week injection cycle, I'd have to give myself a shot every night. In the beginning, my doctors would have to play with the dose to see what I could tolerate—the idea being, the more I could handle, the better—but once they got that right, I shouldn't have too many problems, she said. Except for the fact that I'd have a needle full of chemo waiting for me when I came home from work every day, I thought. My life would be nicely broken up into two-week intervals. Two weeks that I liked and two weeks that I disliked. Oh well. Maybe at the end of all this I'd be cured, I thought. Oh wait, I definitely *wouldn't* be cured. That much I knew. But maybe I'd do really well on the trial, get to remission, or whatever. OK, it was something to shoot for.

Being in a clinical trial was serious business. For me it was more about getting well than contributing to the future of CML treatment, but I couldn't forget that I was a part of medical science, a guinea pig of sorts. Sure, the FDA had already approved both the drugs I'd be taking, so it wasn't exactly a risky, groundbreaking experiment (I wouldn't have done it if it were), but still, I needed to take my role seriously. The trial would last one year and I'd have to keep a very detailed journal throughout the experience. Homework. Each time I came to Oregon, they would go over my entries and we'd discuss everything that was written down. They wanted me to record what time I took my medications each day and document any side effects or other discomfort I was experiencing. They wanted to know about every cough, every bone pain, every headache and stomachache. They did not, however, need to know about hangnails, splinters, chapped lips and the like. Apparently some of the trial participants had been writing memoirs in the lines allotted for ailments and whatever was written down had to be reported. I couldn't help thinking it was like those drug commercials that list 500 side effects including, "in rare cases" blindness, dismemberment, depression and death. Not to worry, I told her. I'd keep it brief. For the trial I would also have to have a blood test once a week for the first six weeks, and then every other week for the duration. Fortunately, I'd be doing that at Sloan. Dr. Cathcart would fax the results to Oregon. She would also do my monthly checkups and consult with Dr. Mauro. I'd be a bicoastal cancer patient. Très chic.

We left the hospital with no drugs—I wasn't allowed to start the trial officially until they had the results of all the blood tests back the next week. Then I'd sign all the paperwork and take my first Gleevec. I'd also learn how to give myself injections. They wanted me to be a pro with a syringe before I left Oregon (and before I started loading it with chemo). In the meantime, we had plenty of things to keep us busy.

It just so happened that while we were out in Portland, some of our family's very best friends, the Cittadinis, were there too. My parents had known Bob and Elizabeth Cittadini forever—my dad and Bob became best friends after they beat the shit out of each other on the first day of 5th grade, and my mom and Elizabeth hit it off as soon as they met and realized they were both dating lunatics. Bob and Elizabeth had four kids—Greg, Jennifer, Kelly and Matt—who my sisters and I basically grew up with. They lived in New Hampshire, but we wrote lots of letters to one another and saw them on holidays and spent summers together, camping out in our backyards and collecting stickers and making up dances. Other than the fact that they said "wicked" a lot and liked Madonna and we said "fresh" and preferred the Beastie Boys, we got along great. We had drifted apart over the years, but we still considered them family. Greg, the oldest son, was now living in Portland with his wife and newborn son (my parents and I had had dinner with them on our first visit). Elizabeth was out in Oregon with Kelly and Jennifer to see the new baby.

At first I was annoyed by the coincidence—I loved the Cittadinis but didn't want to feel obligated to be social. Even 3,000 miles from home, my family had party plans! Plus, I didn't want to crash their little family reunion. But my mom—who was already getting tired of listening to me type—was thrilled to have friends nearby and as soon as I saw them, I was too. Greg cooked us dinner Friday night and Saturday we drove to Cannon beach (I took my laptop with me and banged out a few crucial words in the car on the drive out). We ate fried halibut and drank microbrewery beer and walked along the water. It was spritzing, of course, but the view was still breathtaking. *Goonies* was filmed there—it had those giant rock formations that Sean Astin and the boys lined up in their secret viewfinder—and Nick and I loved that movie. When I called to tell him about it, my mom took a picture of me standing there with my cell phone pressed against my ear. "*What?*" she said, when I looked at her like she was crazy. "You're on one coast, and he's on the other. That's really neat."

On Sunday, Elizabeth and the girls took my mom with them to the Nike headquarters, where Greg worked and where they could shop at the wholesale Nike employee store. I would have loved to go, but instead I stayed at the hotel and worked on my column. I had to email my stuff to Jill on Tuesday morning. She had given me plenty of direction and assured me it would be great, but I was nervous, anxious to let someone read what was going on inside my head. What if she thought I was too candid? Or not candid enough? Or, worse, boring? I was more worried about that than about finally starting the trial. I stayed in my pajamas the whole day, ordered room service and wrote, trying to put the medical stuff in easy-to-understand terms and turning scrambled thoughts into *Glamour*-friendly sentences and paragraphs. And I edited out the abundance of "what the fucks" and "holy shits."

As expected, by Monday all of my blood tests had come back negative (except the one for CML—still had that.) Now all I had to do was learn to wield a syringe. The nurse showed me how to do everything—draw up the liquid, flick the bubbles out of the needle, clean the injection site, and, most importantly, toss the used syringe in a hazardous waste bucket. I loved that I'd be injecting myself with something worthy of being labeled hazardous waste. I spent about half an hour practicing all of that with a syringe full of saline on a fake piece of flesh. My mom snapped pictures the whole time. She documented every event in our lives—big and small—and was never without her camera. My sisters and I usually complained as she ran around at parties and school functions and soccer games saying, "OK, everybody get close" but we loved to look at the photos so we'd smile dutifully and say cheese. With the *Glamour* photographers gone, I was glad she was taking so many pictures. I wanted to be sure we had all the big moments covered for Donald. Plus, I was planning to make a cancer scrapbook.

After becoming a fake-flesh pro, I had to try the shot on myself. At first I didn't trust the nurse that it was OK to inject saline into my body. "Can't this kill me?" I said. "It just seems a little weird, no?" But apparently it was totally fine. I chose my thigh as the site du jour (other popular sites include the belly and the back of the arm, but the latter requires someone else to do it for you—and unless that person was a nurse, no thank you). After my mom's tenth "one, two, three" I stabbed the needle into my leg. "Oh, fuck that hurt," I said as it went in. Dr. Mauro, who was in the room doing paperwork, spun around and said, "Uh-oh." I apologized for my mouth. I could only imagine what these nice Oregon folks thought of me with my four-letter words and my photographers and my cell phone going off every five minutes. Crazy New Yorker, I'm sure. But Dr. Mauro just laughed. I really think he liked me. I wondered if he had as much fun with his other patients as he seemed to have with me. I secretly hoped I would become his favorite.

With the needle still stuck in my leg, I had to push in all the liquid. This is supposed to take seconds. For me, it took minutes. About five of them. It stung so badly and I just couldn't voluntarily hurt myself like that. When I was finally done, I threw the syringe into the waste bucket and everyone clapped. I lied and said, "Piece of cake." I honestly didn't know if I'd be able to handle the real thing, but I didn't want the nurse to make me do it again.

Next on the agenda was swallowing my first Gleevec. For the trial, I'd get the pills for free from the government, (I'd have to pay for the Ara-C on my own). My mom said, "Say cheese," as I put the orange capsules on my tongue and took a big swig of water. "Theeeeese," I said. I was a little embarrassed when my mom asked Dr. Mauro and the nurse to get in the photo, but I knew I'd be glad to have it in my scrapbook. The pills went down without a problem. I kept waiting to throw up or break out in hives, but I never did. Not yet anyway. Dr. Mauro said that the muscle cramping, bone pain and "possible swelling" probably wouldn't kick in for a few days. I'd have to write it all down when it did happen, he reminded me. I signed some paperwork that basically said I wouldn't sue if I did, in fact, grow a third arm, and it was official. I was a part of the clinical trial, patient 007. My mom thought this was the neatest thing ever and took a picture of me holding my patient registration form. Though I didn't get quite the kick out of it that she did, I supposed of all the number patients to be, 007 was pretty cool.

Since we didn't have to be back at the hospital until the

following Monday—for my last tests and to check on how I was tolerating the Gleevec—my mom and I decided we'd drive up to Vancouver and spend a few days there. I had sent my column to Jill so I was free. We could relax, bond a little maybe. My mom and I had never gotten along exceptionally well. We probably spent more time together than anyone else in my family, mostly because she was always traveling with me to one of my volleyball or soccer tournaments, but there was a bit of a wall between us, friction even. My mom was a commenter—she always had something to say about everything, and she never kept her opinion to herself. She was the first born of four and it showed in her bossy ways, ways that drove me crazy. Melissa, on the other hand, was extremely close to my mom. Too much so if you asked me. For one, Melissa and Ysrael ate dinner at my parents' house almost every night, which meant that she had my mom—and my dad for that matter—telling her how to live her life, how she needed to treat her husband and take care of her car and clean her apartment. Melissa didn't seem to mind (probably because she also brought home her laundry which my mom inevitably would do for her). And she and my mom would talk about *everything*. Melissa actually told my mom about the first time she gave a guy a blow job. Even thinking about it now makes me want to hurl. I respected my mom's opinion on a lot of things, but I just didn't let her into my life as much as Melissa did and I think she sometimes resented that.

One of the fundamental issues between us was food. My mom was overweight and I hated that. It's not that I was embarrassed about the way she looked, I just couldn't understand why she didn't want to be thin. Or at least thinner. She had always been so pretty. As a kid, I used to watch *Summer Rental*, the 1985 John Candy vacation movie, and fantasize about someday being like the daughter in the movie (who, coincidentally, was also in *The Goonies*). She had red hair and I thought she was so cool. And so close to her mom. There was a scene where the two of them were walking together on the beach, in bikinis, laughing and checking out all the cute guys. I had long since gotten over the fact that my mom and I were never going to frolic in our bikinis, but I still wanted her to be healthy, to live forever, to always be around to take care of us. Especially now.

Despite her bad diet, my mom had always exercised. She went to the gym and swam and walked. But lately she had started having knee problems and back problems and couldn't move very fast, and that really bothered me. She was only 52. Grandma Del could run circles around her. Actually, Grandma Del may have been part of the problem from the beginning. It couldn't have been easy for my mom to be the daughter of a former Rockette who, even at 80, would turn down dessert very dramatically saying, "Oh, I couldn't possibly." But as a young woman my mom had a beautiful figure (she thought she was fat, of course, but she wasn't). She didn't start really gaining weight until after Meghan was born. She was a stress eater and with three children and a hard-to-please husband (to whom dinner was a religion), she had plenty of it. The clincher, though, she said, was being in the hospital with me when I had ITP. After that, there was no going back. So it was my fault.

When I was growing up, my mom was always on some diet or another, but she never stuck to them. It really seemed like her weight was a big joke to her. Our cabinets were stocked with silly mugs that said things like, "Fat is beautiful" and "I never met a carbohydrate I didn't like"—that one, I now realize, was ahead of its time. Her favorite, though, was a magnet with a picture of a sheep on it that said, "Ewe's not fat, ewe's fluffy." I didn't find it funny at all. But then I had always been a healthy eater—and a little obsessed with my looks. My mom was a really strong, confident woman and her self-image didn't change just because she was heavier than she should be. I loved her for that, and for passing on that confidence to my sisters and me, but I couldn't help thinking she'd be a lot better off if she lost some weight. It was something I thought about more and more since my diagnosis—how could she not try her hardest to be healthy when she saw what was happening to me?—and I supposed that fueled our disconnect. But every time I tried to talk to her about it, I just sounded like an asshole. And I hated to make my mom feel bad. Since I'd been diagnosed, we'd actually been getting along a lot better. Come to think of it, I'd been getting along with everyone a lot better. Not sure what that says about me. But being with her in Oregon for two weeks eating three meals a day wasn't easy. I had to bite my tongue a lot and I suppose I acted out my anger toward her in other ways, like yelling at her for telling me it was raining again.

On our way to Vancouver we stopped for a night to see my friend Amanda. She was living near Tacoma, Washington, with her fiance who was an Army Ranger. Amanda and I had been close friends since we were in elementary school, so to see her cooking Shake 'n Bake chicken while the man she was about to marry polished his boots in the kitchen was a little bizarre. He was preparing to be deployed any day, so it was a bit depressing. Their wedding was planned for August—I was a bridesmaid—and Amanda had no idea when he'd be back. She had no idea where he was going or when she'd be able to talk to him either. She acted very strong, but I knew it couldn't be easy for her. We had a really nice visit with them, but as we said our good-byes I couldn't help thinking that it might be easier to have cancer than to be a military wife.

Vancouver was OK. It rained the whole time, naturally, which was only mildly disappointing since we didn't really feel like doing much of anything anyway. There was a Salvatore Ferragamo store right outside of our hotel and at first I thought I really wanted to buy a bag. My Coach bag was getting old already and I thought it would be so cool to own a Ferragamo bag. But then I realized A: Even in Canadian dollars I couldn't afford a Ferragamo bag and B: I couldn't pull it off. Despite my high-end taste, I wore mostly Gap jeans and Banana Republic shirts. Not exactly haute couture. Instead I bought a Roots T-shirt for Nick and called it a day. My mom and I mostly just emailed people back home and went out to nice dinners—the food in the Pacific Northwest is incredible—and watched On Demand movies in our hotel room. We did take a day trip to Vancouver Island, which probably would have been very beautiful had it not been pouring and had there not been a political protest going on in the streets. We were ready to get back to Portland and back to business.

OHSU has a really great service that allows patients to stay at nearby hotels for free while they're having treatment. Of course you don't get to pick your hotel, but hey, you're not paying. For the first part of the trip, we were in the Doubletree Suites, which was nice, but if you wanted to go downtown you had to take the MAX. The MAX is Portland's public transportation system and it scared the shit out of us. The one time we ventured onto it, there was a young kid flashing a knife to his friend. That was the thing about the city of Portland—it was beautiful and clean and well run, but there was an abundance of derelict kids hanging around. On almost every street corner you could see a kid about my age, who—apart from too many tattoos—looked perfectly healthy and normal, begging for money. It was very strange.

Fortunately, when we got back to Portland, we stayed at the Hilton right smack in the middle of downtown. It was still raining, but we were within walking distance of Saks and Tiffany and the movie theater. We saw *Black Hawk Down* and *40 Days, 40 Nights* and I actually cried more watching the stupid Josh Hartnett movie than I did watching the sad Josh Hartnett movie (though seeing all the hot soldiers die made me feel even worse for Amanda). It depressed me to see a bunch of people my age who were totally carefree, whose only real dilemma was juggling their dates with their drinking and partying. I was jealous, really. No matter what happened from here on out, I no longer didn't have a care in the world. And I really didn't know if I still had my whole life ahead of me to do whatever I wanted with it.

I also didn't know what my family was going to have to deal with next. At first I felt that my getting cancer was like taking one for the team, like maybe we'd be left alone for a while. But it didn't work that way. A week after I was diagnosed, my 27-year-old cousin found out she had multiple sclerosis. Then Grandma Ruth slipped and fell and wound up in the hospital for a month. It seemed unfair, but life was going on for better *and* worse. Nothing could surprise us now, I thought. If I could be told I had cancer at 23 when I was perfectly healthy, anything was possible.

Before we left Portland—and the no sales tax—I had to get Meghan a bone marrow present. (I'd promised to buy something special for whoever was the match.) When I talked to Meghan's roommate, Caroline, a few weeks earlier she told me that Meghan had said that her life had meaning now. That was so nice, and so sad at the same time. But her giving me her marrow would be the ultimate payback. I had bailed Meghan out of so many jams in her lifetime—I hid bad report cards and kept quiet about speeding tickets and bought her beer when she needed it—that I'd given up counting. While she was on her sophomore spring break in South Padre Island, Texas, she called me at work hysterical. She had lost her wallet and it was only the first day of break. She needed me to Western Union her some money immediately. I spent the next few hours locating a Western Union and figuring out exactly how I was going to give her money that I didn't really have. When I called her later that afternoon to say that I had everything all set and I was about to send the money, she said, "Oh, wait. I must have forgotten to call you. I went out to the car and my wallet was wedged between the seats. Isn't that great?"

That was Meghan for you. I really hoped that she'd figure

out what she wanted to do with herself. In the meantime, though, it was pretty cool for her to think that someday she might be able to give her sister life. We could all be on *Oprah*, I thought. Meghan could give me her bone marrow and Melissa could carry my babies. We'd be the redheaded freak family. After spending about three hours in Tiffany—and shamelessly checking out the engagement rings—I finally decided on a sterling silver necklace that had an interlocking knot. It was absolutely perfect. I bought one for myself too so that we'd have matching mementos of our matching marrow.

My last appointment at OHSU was really just a formality. They took more blood, put me on the scale *again* and gave me a prescription for some nausea pills, just in case. Dr. Mauro was excited because another woman from the trial, patient 001 (also very cool) was at the hospital that day and he really wanted us to meet. She was in her late 60s and had started the trial about six months before me. We chatted for a while about the treatment and the side effects. She told me that she hadn't given up her vodka, which I loved to hear. Maybe I will go back to a dirty martini every once in a while, I thought. She also told me that the injections weren't so bad—then she added, sheepishly, that her husband was a doctor and he had been giving her the shots. Cheater. After a while, we started talking about how crazy it was to have such a crazy disease. "I just became a grandmother," she said. "I'm not ready to leave this world. I have so much more life to live." I agreed with her, but couldn't help thinking that she got to be a wife and a mother *and* a grandmother and I was none of those. She had more than 40 years on me. C'mon. If anyone has more life to live, it's *me*. But after spending a little more time with her and seeing photos of her family and hearing her elaborate plans for retirement, I realized that it doesn't matter who or what you are, if you're 22 or 72. Cancer always sucks and you're always too young to have it.

By the end of March, we had advance copies of the May

issue with my first column in it. It had taken a few revisions to get it just right, but Cindi was really pleased. And she pretty much let me say whatever I wanted, including one holy shit. I even got a line on the cover: "Cancer at 23: A *Glamour* staffer shares her battle to live." By that point it was pretty clear to everyone that I was going to live, at least for a while, so it was a little weird to see such a dramatic headline, but I suppose I understood. "Cancer at 23: A *Glamour* staffer maintains a normal life" wouldn't exactly fly off the shelves. So a battle it was.

6 Cancer becomes my second job

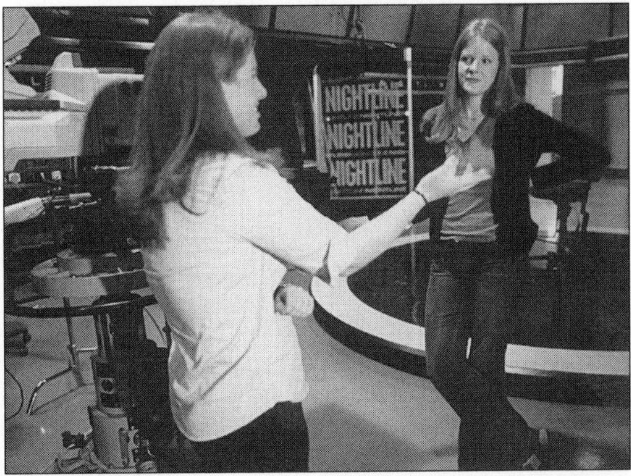

Preparing for my Nightline *interview*

I MAY HAVE MISSED THE DUNGENESS CRAB, THE FULL Sail beer and the maid service, but I was happy to be back on the East Coast. It was great to see everyone, especially Nick and my dad, who admitted they had been a little lost without their women. It was even good to be back at the office, plugged in again. Whenever I was away from the pod for too long I felt out of touch with the world—mostly the world of *The Bachelor, Sex and the City* and the *New York Post*'s gossip column, Page Six, but still, being back was refreshing. I was starting to experience some bone pain and cramping from the Gleevec, but that was a good thing. Dr. Mauro had told me that it meant that the marrow was active, that the Gleevec was blasting all those bad leukemia cells. I tried to remember that as I attempted to climb stairs or cross my legs or do pretty much anything without screaming out in pain. It was as if I'd just run a marathon. I looked like a 300-year-old woman hobbling around the office. But I wasn't puffy so I really couldn't complain. And Dr. Mauro assured me that the pain would pass.

Meanwhile, I had to start the Ara-C injections. My mom really wanted me to come out to Huntington for the night so she could help me with my first shot, but for the whole week leading up to it I thought it was no big deal. I might need Nick to come to my apartment for moral support, but I could handle the shot no problem. Then, a few hours before I was supposed to do it, I took a closer look in the bag that I had picked up from the Huntington pharmacy. (The pharmacy at Sloan didn't take my insurance.) There were vials of liquid *and* vials of powder, which meant that I would have to mix my own chemo *then* draw it into the syringe *then* stick it into myself. But that hadn't been part of the dress rehearsal at OHSU. Shit. I called my trial nurse who said that some pharmacies just do it that way. It wasn't ideal but it was fine; I'd just have to follow the instructions.

This I could not handle. I hung up and hopped on a train to Huntington.

Always thinking, my mom had called her friend Randy, a nurse, to come to the house to help us. For once, I didn't mind having a houseguest on a Tuesday night. When Randy arrived, the place was a zoo. My dad was frantically searching for his reading glasses so he could look at the calculator he was using to try to figure out how many ccs I'd need to equal 12 milliliters, I was telling Nick that I had to be careful not to have bubbles in the syringe or I could die, and my mom was rifling through the kitchen drawers for film for her camera. When she finally found it, she took a picture of Randy reading the chemo instructions and my dad said, "Jesus Christ, Cindy, put that thing away." The tension was so thick you could pierce it with one of the 14 syringes spread across the kitchen counter. Poor Randy.

Finally, we—and by we I mean Randy—figured out the right ratio. But the problem wasn't completely solved. The stupid pharmacy had given us the wrong size syringes, so she had to fill two to get me the right dose. Two shots! I didn't sign up for that. But I had to play it cool because my parents looked like they were about to cry. Randy did the first one in my arm and I did the other in my thigh. As I pulled the needle out of my leg, my dad said, "Who needs a martini?" I opted for New York Super Fudge Chunk ice cream and went into the living room with Nick and his martini to watch TV. Again, we waited for me to pass out or start convulsing, but nothing. The effects of Ara-C are cumulative, so I would probably start feeling something—nausea, fatigue—about a week into the injection cycle. I couldn't wait. Randy had tried to teach me how to measure out the powder and the liquid, but I knew I could never do it that way again.

As it turned out, the injections from Sloan only cost $60 a month and came in ready-to-use pre-filled syringes that you keep in the refrigerator. My mom and I agreed that when it came to cancer, it just wasn't worth trying to save money and the next day I picked up the 13 remaining shots from Sloan. It was the best $60 I'd ever spent.

With my treatment fully underway, I went to my first official cancer meeting. It was at the Leukemia & Lymphoma Society but it was far from a support group. Before I left for Oregon I had done a little Net surfing on my disease, checking out all the websites I had previously been too afraid to look at. On the Leukemia & Lymphoma Society site, I saw a listing for a fundraising golf tournament with the Yankees. My family are huge Mets fans, not Yankees fans, but we do love golf and I thought the event would make great fodder for my next column. Not to mention awesome photos for Donald. I clicked on the icon for more info. Since I was writing about leukemia for a huge national magazine, I figured I could get press passes, put together a Zammett family foursome.

I called the contact person from the website and introduced myself. Her name was Leslie and she was just about the nicest woman I'd ever talked to. We chatted for a long time about my diagnosis and my treatment and my column. Unfortunately the golf tournament had been cancelled—between September 11 and the economy, they just didn't have the money to do it this year, she said. I was bummed and almost got off the phone with her, but then she told me about a bunch of other things they had going on. The society had a young professionals group called Society Ties that raised funds by hosting bar parties and casino nights and stuff like that. They were preparing for a big event called The Man and Woman of the Year and she would love to have me come to the next committee meeting to learn more about it. I hadn't really thought about getting *that* involved—really, I just wanted to meet Derek Jeter—but I told her I'd come to the meeting and check it out.

I was so nervous I almost didn't show up. I knew that we'd have to go around the room and introduce ourselves and tell everyone why we were there and I was dreading it. Most people in the group had some connection to a blood-related cancer—a grandmother who had died, a friend who had beat it—but I was a *patient*. When my turn came, my stomach was at my feet and my voice came out all quivery. "I'm Erin Zammett, I work at *Glamour* magazine and I'm here because four months ago I was diagnosed with chronic myelogenous leukemia, or CML. But I'm taking really good drugs so I'm not sick and I wanted to get involved." It was still a little hard to say all of that out loud.

After that awkward AA beginning, the meeting got down to business. The Man and Woman of the Year contest was about to start. It was a six-week long fundraising competition where candidates do whatever they can—write letters, throw parties, have bowl-athons—to raise money for the Society. The male candidate who raises the most becomes the Man of the Year, and the female candidate who raises the most is named Woman of the Year. The winners get a bunch of nice prizes, their names in *USA Today* and a video about them played on the Jumbotron in

Times Square. But, Leslie stressed, it's not about the prizes. It's about helping to improve patients' lives.

The LLS, as everyone in the know calls it, funds research for blood-related cancers (leukemia, lymphoma, myeloma), specifically for the development of new drugs. In fact, the Society had given millions to Dr. Druker to support his Gleevec research and was continuing to support his efforts to make the drug even more efficient. In addition to advancing the future of cancer treatment, the Society also gives money to patients to help with medical expenses (the maximum reimbursement is $500, which I can tell you doesn't scratch the surface, but still, it's something). And it holds seminars and support groups to help patients and their families feel more informed and less alone.

I hadn't really done much volunteer work since high school and even then it was fueled by my desire to look well-rounded on my college applications—and because all the cool kids did Key Club. I just didn't think I had the time for charity work (I did, however, have the time to watch about two hours of TV a night). And I didn't feel completely attached to any one cause. But all of that was about to change. Sitting in that meeting made me realize that I could do something good with my diagnosis, that I had the opportunity to help others and by doing so, help myself. When we were younger my friends and I would cut through the woods in back of Lucy's house sometimes. We'd all be totally freaked out, but I'd have to pretend not to be. I was the tallest in the group so I was often looked upon as the leader. I had to be strong for the others, so I'd skip ahead, tell them that there was nothing to be afraid of. And invariably I'd be less afraid myself. Anything that made me less of a victim was right up my alley. I liked to take action, to be in control. I figured if I couldn't do something good with my diagnosis, I'd just be a sad, scared cancer patient, and that was the last thing I wanted to be. Plus, all the partying sounded like a lot of fun.

About a week later, I went to a Society Ties bar fundraiser. I brought a bunch of friends from work, who were more than happy to pay the five-dollar cover and drink for a cause. It was really fun to be out at happy hour with a bunch of cool, young people drinking and partying and raising money. I blended in so well that they probably just assumed I was another volunteer. Part of me wanted to tell them all that I had leukemia—to see their reaction, to hear them say, "*Really*? You don't look sick at all." Cancer made me feel special in a weird way, but it was about more than getting attention. I just didn't see the point of *not* telling people. I didn't feel bad for myself and I didn't want other people to either. But instead of playing show and tell with my bottle of Gleevec, I had a pint of Bass Ale. And then another. I got a little righteous, thinking, I'm 24, I live in Manhattan, I should be doing shots of tequila not shots of chemo. Bartender, gimme another. But I hadn't eaten dinner so the beers went right to my head. On my way home I stopped at the Chinese Mexican place next to my building and picked up a bean burrito, which I scarfed down so I'd have something other than alcohol in my stomach before doing my injection. It was too little too late. I woke up three times in the middle of the night to puke my guts out. Damn it. It was only my first round of injections and already I'd blown it. I could almost hear the cancer gods saying, "Psst, remember us?"

But it may not have been completely the beer's fault. As it turned out, the Ara-C dose they started me on was way too high. Even when I hadn't just had a frosty beverage, I started to really feel like I was on chemo, or what I had imagined being on chemo would feel like. I got nauseated easily and my energy was completely zapped. Some days it seemed like I was walking through quicksand. It wasn't just hard to get out of bed in the morning, it was hard to walk the two blocks to the subway and to sit at my desk and to pick up the phone. But I would have grinned and beared all of that had the shots not also affected my neutrophils, the blood cells that keep me from getting sick. When that count fell too low—which it did several times—I had to stop the shots until it stabilized again.

I didn't mind the break from the injections, of course, but it seemed a little like cheating. Sure, I hated stabbing myself with needles, but I had accepted that that was part of the plan and I wanted to stick with the protocol that was supposed to make me better. It was one of the many cancer Catch-22s I experienced, kind of like when my high school soccer coach would tell the team we didn't have to run sprints that day at practice. We'd all say, "Thanks Coach, you're the best!" and high-five each other because, let's face it, sprints suck. But deep down we'd know we really needed the speed and agility that those sprints gave us if we were going to win the big game on Saturday. And beating cancer was a little more important than beating the Northport Tigers. I wanted to do whatever it took. I didn't want any breaks. And I couldn't help thinking that the more the treatment hurt me, the more it was working.

For the first two months of the trial, I was at Sloan almost every other day for blood tests. At one point my counts got so low that I had to stop both the shots *and* the Gleevec. Dr. Cathcart told me to avoid eating at salad bars and buffets. Apparently there are a lot of germs lurking in food that sits out all day and my immune system wasn't quite up to fighting whatever the sneeze guard didn't catch. Considering I got my lunch from the Condé Nast cafeteria salad bar almost every day, I found this information disheartening—and disgusting. I'd never look at shredded carrots and three bean salad the same way again, neutrophils or no neutrophils.

The constant stopping and starting was frustrating, but eventually we got the dose right and my treatment became a bit more streamlined. I only had to go to Sloan once every two weeks. By this point the bone pain and cramping from the Gleevec had subsided and though I still dragged a little during the injection cycles and had to pop the occasional anti-nausea pill, the side effects weren't nearly as bad as they'd been in the beginning. Of course, as my luck would have it, the two-week cycle we finally settled on coincided with my period—I'd get it one week into the injections, when the effects from the Ara-C were just kicking in. I had never been completely crippled by my period like some women are, but adding chemo and needles to cramps and mood swings wasn't pleasant. I dreaded the shots—both the act of giving them and the side effects they produced—so much that it depressed me. For the first and only time during my life with cancer, I felt bad for myself.

In the meantime, I decided to nominate Melissa for the Man and Woman of the Year competition. I could have been the candidate myself, but I knew it would have felt too weird to ask people for money for a disease that I had—what if they said no? This way, Melissa could raise the money in my honor and I could help out behind the scenes. Besides, I knew Melissa would take it seriously. She loved money (even if it wasn't money she'd get to keep) and she was super competitive. About 15 years earlier when we were fishing on my parents' boat, my dad's friend Bob Melillo (most of my dad's friends are named Bob) told me he'd give me $5 if I ate one of the little bait fish we had caught. Though my dad was cheering me on and the thing was dead and only about two-inches long, I chickened out. Melissa, whose ears perked up as soon as she heard the challenge, dropped her fishing pole, walked to the bucket of fish, looked at Bob, said, "Five bucks, right?" and swallowed it. I thought she was crazy—and kind of cool. She was just happy to be five dollars richer than me. My dad always said that Melissa was his "son." She screamed at the TV during Mets games, ate steak rare, drank beer, cursed like a sailor, loved to gamble and ate bait for cash. I knew with her at the helm we could outraise anyone.

The competition kicked off on April 29 and would end on June 12. We figured we could raise at least $10,000 in the six-week period. We recruited Jaimee and my roommate, Karen, to help and started by each sending a letter to every person we knew—telling my story, explaining how the Leukemia & Lymphoma Society helps people like me and asking for donations. We stuck a photocopy of my first column, "Cancer at 23," in each envelope to drive home our point. Within two days of our big mailing, the money started pouring in. Ever since I'd been diagnosed our friends and family had been asking what they could do for me, but there really wasn't anything I needed, especially since I was never actually sick. It was just another of the many ways that cancer makes the people around it feel completely helpless. But now there was something for everyone to do. They could donate to our campaign and feel like they were making a difference for me—and for others. And as I was quickly learning, that felt really good.

Soon, Melissa and I were completely consumed by the competition. Every day we'd send new checks to the LLS so they could add them to our total. We were constantly touching base with each other, cooking up new ways to raise more money, strategizing how we would beat the other candidates. I went to Huntington every weekend to make calls and secure auction prizes for the fundraising parties we were planning. At some points, we actually had to remind ourselves that it was all for a good cause and that there was no reason to lose sleep over the font for the donation letters. We just really wanted to win. I think both of us felt that in some ways the more money we raised, the better I'd do on my treatment, like it was a penance of sorts, though as far as I knew getting cancer wasn't a sin. Whatever the reason, we were out for blood (no pun intended), and we were having a blast.

A few weeks into the competition, *Glamour* hosted a party for us—a two-hour open bar at The Bryant Park Hotel. Because the magazine was picking up the tab for the space and liquor, every penny of the $20 cover went to the LLS. Over 200 people showed up—at one point, the line to get in stretched around the block. Publicists I'd talked to on the phone but never met in person were there, guys from high school who were too-cool seniors when I was a freshman came and partied, girls from my old volleyball team drove in from Long Island to show their support. It was hard to comprehend that they were all there for me. Since joining the LLS and becoming so immersed in the fundraising, I had kind of forgotten that I was still a patient. Most of the time I felt like I was just another volunteer raising money for a good cause. But that night, as I looked around at the packed room, I remembered that it wasn't just a good cause, it was *my* cause. At the end of the two hours we had raised over $9000. We had almost reached our goal in one night. And we weren't stopping there. We wanted to raise twice that much, to double our goal, to squash the competition. But first I had some business to take care of.

A few days after the party, I headed back out to Oregon with my mom for a biopsy that would tell us if the drugs were working (Melissa held down the fort at fundraising central). The photographers didn't join us this time, which was a huge bonus. I really liked John and his assistant, but there was something not quite right about showing up for a bone marrow biopsy in full makeup with blown-out hair, mugging for the camera. I wanted to keep the visit simple, to get in, get out and go hit the outlet stores. Portland had a big, gorgeous outdoor outlet mall with a Banana Republic and a Ralph Lauren and huge discounts. And if we went while I was still limping from my biopsy, my mom would feel so bad she wouldn't let me pay for anything. The best discount of all.

The visit would have been completely uneventful had it not been for Mark, the eccentric, bluegrass-singing nurse. Mark was something of a mascot at OHSU. He was really tall and really thin and rode a scooter to work, which couldn't have been easy since OHSU sat on top of a massive hill (with amazing views of Mt. Hood on clear days). He wore Birkenstocks and Hawaiian shirts and looked kind of like Jimmy Buffett. I first met him in the blood-draw room in the brand new bone marrow transplant and leukemia wing at OHSU. The room was set up like a hair salon, minus the mirrors and shampoo sinks. The nurses actually reminded me of hairdressers too, as they bustled around from station to station, chatting loudly with each other and making small talk with the patients—patients who looked far worse off than me.

"You get Ativan, right?" Mark said as he sidled up to my chair and clamped a bag to an IV pole. "No," I said. "I've never had it." Apparently, most patients who are going in for a biopsy get the drug to calm their nerves before the procedure. I explained to him that I'd already had a biopsy with Dr. Mauro—sans drugs—and survived just fine. And that I'd rather have a little discomfort for 20 minutes than walk around in a drugged-up fog for the whole day. "Okey dokey," he said, and wheeled the stuff away. The nurses who were milling around seemed impressed, shocked even, that I didn't take the drug. At least none of them did the little, "Wow, aren't you brave!" routine that just made me feel patronized. Mark said that since I wasn't getting the Ativan, he'd come into the exam room with me and sing some of his new songs. It'd be as good as drugs, he promised. No thank you! I didn't want this kooky man in the room while I had a giant needle screwed into my back. But I couldn't tell him no. He was way too excited.

Just as Dr. Mauro was about to start numbing the biopsy site on my hipbone, Mark moseyed into the room with a ukelele in his hand and a harmonica dangling from his neck. "You didn't forget about me, did ya?" he said. Within seconds Mark became a one-man band, strumming and humming and singing songs he seemed to make up as he went along. One was about a Mac computer breaking down, one was about a porta potty falling off a pick-up truck, one was about unrequited love. At first I just wanted him to stop—I felt embarrassed and uncomfortable about the whole thing. But then I got over being such a stick in the mud and figured what the hell. It was better than having my picture taken and his lyrics were actually really good. And I needed the distraction—this biopsy wasn't quite as painless as the last one. I felt a lot of the twisting and pushing. I tried to focus on Mark's melodies instead of the pain, but right at the end of the procedure it felt like the needle had plunged straight through my bone and out the other side. I screamed, "Fuck!" which put a bit of a damper on the whole campfire thing we had going on. Mark decided to take five.

Unfortunately we wouldn't get the results from the biopsy for about three weeks. From what they could see from the many blood tests I'd had during the dosing debacle, everything was going as planned. Still, I couldn't help thinking about what we'd do if the Gleevec wasn't working—and there was a one in five chance that it wouldn't be. What would we do if it worked a little but not as much as we'd hoped for? Would I go right to transplant or give the drug another 12 weeks to work? Of course there was absolutely nothing I could do to help the odds turn in my favor—no wheat germ shake to drink, no yoga position to try, no extra assignment to bring up my grade. I'd just have to sit back and hope. That was still the hardest part about having cancer. I had no control over it.

What I did have control over was our fundraising. And I was getting good at it. When I got back to New York, the competition was picking up serious steam—our total was up to almost $20,000. With about a week left to go, we threw a big party in Huntington at a cool new restaurant called Blue Honu. We had food and an open bar and door prizes and an awesome silent auction table. My second column had just come out so we had a bunch of issues strewn around for people to take. Unlike the *Glamour* party, we had to get everything donated, but that was half the fun. The guys at Blue Honu were more than generous and pretty much gave us the space and appetizers for free. Melissa and my mom hit up local venders for gift certificates, and I used my *Glamour* contacts to put together awesome baskets of best-selling books and jewelry and beauty products. A girl Melissa and I had gone to high school with worked as an alcohol sales rep and took care of all the beer and vodka and gin—the most important stuff.

Coors had even made us a huge banner to hang outside the restaurant that said, "A Leukemia & Lymphoma Society Fundraiser in Honor of Erin Zammett." I was so excited to put it up—it was like having my name on the marquee, I was a cancer star!—but as we unraveled the sign, we realized that it said "Leukemia & *Lump*homa Society." Whoops. At first I was laughing about the typo, but then I started to get upset. Then I refused to hang up the sign. I was a journalist, how could a sign at my party be spelled wrong? Just as I was about to roll it back up, my mom, the regulator, came outside. "Who the hell is gonna notice that?" she said. "It's not like anyone at the party has lymphoma and even if they did, they probably wouldn't notice." She told me to calm down and go inside. She'd have Ysrael run to the stationery store around the corner to get a marker and they'd draw a tail on the U. "You'll never even know the difference," she said. "Fine," I huffed and went to arrange the auction table. At least leukemia was spelled right.

In the end, of course, it didn't matter what the sign said—or that the makeshift Y looked a lot worse than the U. The night was perfect. We had a huge turnout, everyone had a great time and when the party was over, we had raised $14,000. A lot of people run races for charity or do walks or sell T-shirts, but in my family, partying was clearly the way to go.

I was sitting at my desk at *Glamour* when Dr. Mauro called with the results from my biopsy. The second I saw the 503 area code pop up on my caller ID I felt like I was going to puke. "I have some good news," he said right away, knowing I'd be anxious. "Only four percent of your cells are showing leukemia right now—that's down from 98 percent when you were diagnosed. You've had a remarkable response." The drugs were working. I was so relieved I started crying. Then Dr. Mauro explained what all of this meant in the big picture, something I was increasingly interested in seeing. There were three types of response—hematological (no evidence in blood cell numbers), cytogenetic (no evidence in the chromosomes of cells) and molecular (no evidence in the DNA). I had already had a hematological response on the hydroxurea. That was easy. What we were going for with the trial was cytogenetic remission—meaning no sign of leukemia in any of my cells. Doctors believed that patients who got to this point would have a much greater chance of staying in remission than those who still had some disease lurking around—even, say, four percent. The ultimate goal of Gleevec, the Holy Grail if you will, was to get patients to molecular response, achieving something called "complete molecular remission," but we'd discuss that down the road. First, we had to get that four percent down to zero.

"Has anyone ever gotten to zero in the first three months?" I couldn't help asking. Of course I was happy with my response, but it wasn't perfect. It reminded me of when I'd come home from school with a 97 on a test and my dad would say, only half-joking, "what happened to the other three points?" Dr. Mauro told me that yes, there were some patients who got down to undetectable levels in three months. I hated those patients. Then he assured me that I was definitely in the top percent of patient response and that he had no reason to think that I wouldn't get to cytogenetic remission. He also mentioned, in his cover-all-the-bases, doctorly way, that there are some patients who have a big response at first, but then plateau. In other words, I wasn't in the clear yet. But before we hung up, Dr. Mauro told me that he was thrilled with my progress. "Go celebrate," he said. Not being one to count my cancer cells before they hatch, I decided to keep my celebrating low key—take-out sushi and *The Bachelor.*

At the end of June, Melissa was named Woman of the Year for The Leukemia & Lymphoma Society. We had raised $36,000, a record for the New York City chapter. At the awards party, we were giddy, so relieved that we made it, so proud of our accomplishment (and so excited we'd get to star in the LLS promo on the Jumbotron). It was an emotional night—both because our epic fundraising journey had come to a dramatic end and because there was no Beefeater gin for my dad's martini and only crudités and chips and salsa for him to eat. We partied nonetheless and before the night ended, I had my first taste of fame. As Karen, Jaimee, Melissa and I posed for pictures with the Man of the Year and his team, I noticed two girls staring at me and whispering to each other. When the pictures were finally over, the girls walked up to me slowly, and very cautiously one of them said, "Are you the girl that writes for *Glamour*?" I've been recognized! "I am," I said, and introduced myself. She looked at the other girl and said, "See! I knew it." They had read the first two installments of my cancer diary and loved them and couldn't wait for the third. I felt like a celebrity—a cancerlebrity anyway.

I'd actually been getting quite a bit of attention since my first column hit newsstands.

I started receiving letters and emails from readers almost immediately. They came from fellow CML patients and family members of patients and people with other types of cancers and even perfectly healthy readers. At first I was shocked by the response. When you sit in front of a computer all day, it's easy to forget that there's a whole country out there reading the magazine you're producing. My words were reaching millions of people each month, a fact that still blows me away. A lot of the letters were tough to get through—one was from a mother whose only child had CML before the days of Gleevec and didn't survive. But even the happy ones made me cry. Every one thanked me for sharing my story, for making them feel less alone, for giving them hope. They told me they would pray for me and run marathons for me. One woman even told me she'd take me shopping the next time I was in Portland. It's not that my other *Glamour* stories, things with titles like, "Hey Guys, What Were You Thinking about the Last Time You Had Sex?" weren't important to our readers, but this was different. This was my *life*. And to be able to do something so positive with such a negative part of that life, to know that my experience might be helping someone, was an incredible feeling. I wrote back to almost every person who wrote me (give or take a few of the inevitable weird ones) and saved every email and letter I received. Even the ones from prison.

A few newspapers interviewed me about my life with cancer, which was pretty cool. It was fun to read about my experience in someone else's words—and it gave my mom more material for my baby book: "Baby's first cancer press." Then *Nightline* did a half-hour special on me, which was totally crazy. One of the researchers for the show was flipping through a May *Glamour* and came across my first column. She had red hair and a close family just like me and felt an instant connection. She wanted to profile me—my diagnosis, the trial, what it was like to write about my cancer in a huge national magazine. Her producer thought it was a good idea, too. So did *Glamour*. I had to do extensive phone interviews so they could make sure I was comfortable talking about everything and, I presume, to see if I was articulate enough for national television. I passed the test and right before the Fourth of July I went to Washington, D.C., for the interview. Amy Peck, *Glamour*'s publicist and one of my favorite people at the magazine, came along to coach me and to keep me calm and to make sure the *Nightline* people showed a cover of *Glamour* in one of the shots. All of the attention I was getting for my column was good for the magazine, and they encouraged me to do as much publicity as possible. I was happy to do it. I was truly indebted to Cindi for giving me the opportunity to share my experience with our readers. Writing the column was my therapy—and the people I met and heard from and interacted with as a result were my support group. Of course the *Glamour* photographer came with us to D.C., which was kind of annoying and kind of embarrassing. I didn't want Ted Koppel to think I was a diva, which, when you travel with your own photographer and publicist, is a tough label to avoid. But in a way I loved having my entourage.

As embarrassing as it is to admit, I had always wanted to be a little famous. My college friends like to remind me that I used to tell people I would be on *Letterman* by the time I was 25. Though I do remember saying that, I really think it was more of a defense mechanism than anything else. If life was sucking, or a teacher gave me a hard time or some guy I liked brushed me off, I'd think to myself, "If they only knew how great I'm going to be." I'd picture the asshole guy lying in bed one night, beer can resting on beer belly, flipping through the channels and there I'd be making small talk with Dave. I loved that fantasy. And I guess after a few too many amaretto sours (my drink of choice sophomore year, don't ask), I shared that fantasy with anyone who would listen.

I also used to practice my Oscar acceptance speech in the shower. I didn't want to be an actress, mind you. And I wasn't really interested in being a screenplay writer at that point, though now it sounds like a fun gig. I just wanted to be good enough at something that people—*a lot* of people—would notice. It's not that original a dream, but I wanted to have an impact on the world. So it was Ted Koppel instead of David Letterman, and cancer instead of whatever non life-threatening thing I would have preferred to be getting interviewed about. It was still pretty cool. And I wasn't 25 yet.

And that wasn't all. A few weeks after the *Nightline* interview, the video of Melissa and me was running on the Jumbotron in Times Square. A videographer had come out to Huntington to capture us "in our own environment." We went out on my dad's boat and talked and posed and giggled, desperately trying to act natural. It wound up being just a 15-second spot, but it was great. They had edited it to be a close up of Melissa and me looking out into the sunset, then turning to face each other, brushing the hair out of our eyes and smiling in a carefree, sisterly way. The LLS info ran across the bottom of the screen, telling people how and why to donate money.

It was pretty cool to be standing in the heart of New York City looking up at my sister and me on the big screen—my mom came in and took pictures of me staring at it—but it was even cooler to know what we had accomplished. To know that we had raised all that money in just six weeks. To know that we could make a difference, that we could make lemonade from lemons. I'm not one of those people who goes around saying, "everything happens for a reason," but I was really starting to feel like this whole cancer thing wasn't for naught. I was using my experience to help others. I suppose it's a little sad to think that it took getting a potentially deadly disease to make me a more giving person, but it was true. My life was getting better, *I* was getting better, since I'd been diagnosed. For so long I talked about how weird it was to have cancer and not have anything change, but the truth was, things were changing. And I was glad.

7 Love sick

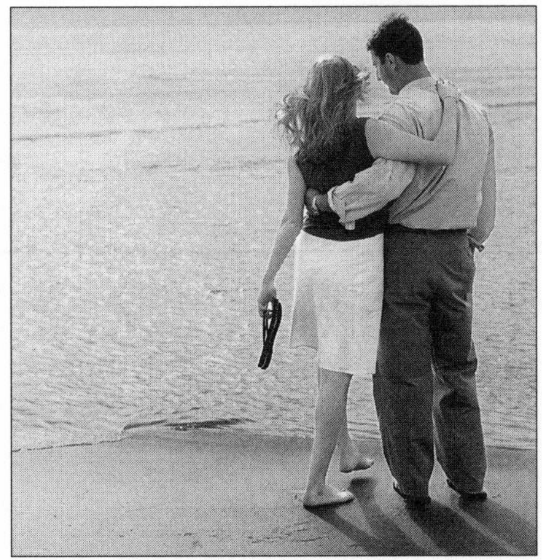

Walking with Nick on the Oregon coast

BACK WHEN I WAS FIRST DIAGNOSED, I HAD THE FLU. IT was totally unrelated to my cancer, but I felt awful nonetheless and spent three days in bed. During that time, Nick was the most caring, attentive and loving I'd ever seen him. He made me soup and got me my medicine and checked on me constantly. He brought me flowers and cleaned my apartment and walked 10 blocks and five avenues to the nearest Blockbuster to rent *The Princess Diaries*—then watched it with me without complaining. It was almost like he had been waiting to have the opportunity to take care of me, to show me how good he could be at it. It made sense too. I had cancer, I *should* be sick and he *should* be taking care of me. But since then there had been very few opportunities for him to play nurse. And the further away we got from my diagnosis, the less sympathy I got. It just wasn't as easy for him to feel bad for me when I was getting up early on the weekends to go to the gym and working late and going to LLS meetings and parties. I had also started writing essays and giving speeches about my experience for various organizations, which made my already packed schedule even crazier. Nick told me that some days he felt more like my assistant or my sidekick than my boyfriend. And he had a point. Because I didn't want to say no to anything, I had spread myself a little thin. I was always running late, always stressing out, always overwhelmed. And my relationship with Nick was the last thing on my to-do list. But if I didn't want to lose him, I'd have to make room for him in my life.

My next bone marrow biopsy—marking six months on the trial—was scheduled for the end of July. Though my mom and I had really started looking forward to our trips together, I decided I should take Nick this time. He could meet Dr. Mauro and see OHSU and feel a little more involved in everything. I also figured it would be good for us to get away, even if it was for cancer, not pleasure. July was one of the few months when it didn't rain in Portland, so we could do some sightseeing, check out the rose gardens and the Columbia River Gorge. My mom was sad she wouldn't be getting her mini-vacation, which is what our trips together had become, but agreed it was a good idea.

Because I had flown to Oregon so many times, I'd become a OnePass elite member on Continental and could upgrade us to first class. This meant that we had lobster appetizers and ice cream sundaes and leg room. This also meant that the alcohol flowed freely from the moment we boarded the plane, a luxury that Nick took full advantage of. By the time we arrived in Portland he'd had one Heineken, three gin and tonics and several glasses of wine. I was a little upset about his overindulgence, but I knew he didn't love to fly and that he was nervous about going with me for the biopsy so I tried not to get mad. But when he rang the flight attendant call button to get yet another refill on his merlot, I couldn't hold my tongue any longer. We were fighting before we even checked in.

As it turned out, my *Nightline* special aired the night we arrived. It didn't come on until midnight Portland time which was 3 a.m. on our body clocks. Being so bleary-eyed made the experience of watching myself on TV even more surreal. I was so weirded out that I couldn't even focus on what I was saying. I thought my voice sounded strange and my face looked fat and I kept wishing they would change the damn camera angle. The whole interview was shot on my bad side, and I was obsessing about a scar to the left of my eye where I had had a mole removed in sixth grade. I really needed to get that fixed.

The next morning, just as we were waking up, Nick's college friend Jeff, whom Nick lovingly called "Turd," arrived into town. He lived about three hours north in Washington State and Nick had kindly invited him to come hang out with us for a day or so, and crash in our hotel room. I was livid when Nick first mentioned this to me a few weeks earlier. It's not like it was our honeymoon, but I was really looking forward to being alone, having some quality time, some sex (doing chemo right before bed hadn't exactly done wonders for my libido and for once I wasn't on my injections). Not to mention that the trip was really about cancer, not fun. But I did understand his dilemma. Jeff was one of his best friends, and he hadn't seen him in almost a year and we were all the way across the country, so close to where he lived. It would have been "so fucked up, Erin" if we didn't tell him we were coming. So, the three of us drove out to the coast (something I tried to do every time I was in Oregon) and ate the fish and chips and drank the microbrewed beer and went for a long walk on the beach. I had a great time, of course, and it was really good to see Jeff, who was one of my favorite of Nick's friends. But that was kind of beside the point.

That night, the three of us went out to dinner back in Portland. We ate more and drank more and talked more. Then we walked back to the hotel and the boys went to the bar, and I went up to the room and watched *Monsters, Inc.* I was sucked into the movie but not enough to keep me from thinking that there I was, the cancer patient, the one whom the trip was about, up in the room all alone watching a cartoon (albeit a really cool digitally animated one). I suppose part of me was just jealous that I couldn't be down at the bar drinking with the boys like I used to be able to do. But another part of me wished I'd brought my mom on the trip. She was always so good to me when we were out there. Sure she told my life story to every concierge and waitress and store clerk we met and dipped her dungeness crab in butter even though it really didn't need it, but she also took really good care of me and I needed that. Even though I was healthy and had a good attitude about my cancer and had adapted well to life with the disease, being in Oregon was still hard. It made the whole thing very real and sometimes I just wanted to be doted on a little and my mom knew that. Nick was still learning.

The boys finally came upstairs at 1 a.m. Nick stumbled into the bed with me and Jeff slept in a cot about a foot away—very romantic. Then they got up at 5:30 a.m., still drunk, to head to the golf course for a "really quick 18." Before they left Nick very dramatically puked his guts out in the bathroom. I stayed in bed late, watched another On Demand movie then went for a walk on the river. When the boys got back, they flopped on the bed, blasted SportsCenter, ordered room service and passed out for three hours. Unable to stand the smell of French fry grease and laziness on a gorgeous day, I went down to the lobby and read for as long as I could before becoming completely annoyed.

When I went back to the room, I could tell Nick was ready for some alone time too. As much as he loved his friends there was only so much boozing and bullshitting he could take before he needed a break. Plus, I knew he wanted to spend time with me. Nick always said that he'd rather do nothing with me than something with anyone else and I believed that. Still, when Jeff left later that afternoon, I made Nick come clothes shopping with me as punishment. Then we went to a great dinner. Nick ordered Osso Buco and ate the marrow in my honor. He told me that no matter how bad things may be, or how bad they may get, they never seem unbearable because he has me. We had a really nice time. But it didn't last.

The next morning I was fighting with Nick before he'd even gotten out of bed. It was the day of my biopsy and John (the *Glamour* photographer) and his assistant were meeting us at the hotel about an hour before the appointment so they could get some casual shots of Nick and me hanging out together. We had woken up early, and I asked Nick if he would come with me for a walk on the river. He was hungry and said he was going to order steak and eggs first. But I was antsy: Couldn't we grab one of those little boxes of cereal from the gift shop to tide us over, then go for a walk, then have a nice breakfast in an actual restaurant instead of in bed (which just seemed lazy to me)? Nope. He was starving. And he wanted steak and eggs. I couldn't help thinking that the reason he wanted room service in the first place was because *Glamour* was paying for the room—since we were shooting in there—and he wanted to take advantage. Nick sometimes had a bit of an entitlement problem. He also hated being told what to do and had grown quite accustomed to getting his way. Growing up, he'd do something bad—like pick up a piece of already chewed bubblegum from the ground and stick it in his little sister's mouth—get punished for it, then cry until his mom revoked the punishment, which she always did. I loved his mom but she had created a bit of a monster. He wanted steak and eggs and he was going to get it, *now*.

We argued in circles for a few minutes, then I stormed out of the room, called Melissa from my cell and cried to her for my whole 40-minute walk. We agreed that I was a crazy micromanager, and I should let him eat breakfast and order whatever he wants and not read into it like he's making some grand statement by getting the most expensive thing on the menu. But we also agreed that as the patient on the day of my biopsy I should be able to be as crazy as I wanted to be—and the asshole should have gotten his lazy ass out of bed and gone for a fucking walk with me. Armed with this theory, I went back to the room. And things got worse. I couldn't find anything to wear. I felt fat and ugly and the photographers were on their way to our hotel room—not to mention I had the weigh-in to look forward to, which is probably where the first flip-out had stemmed from (how can I eat a huge breakfast before getting on a scale?)

Nick tried to calm me down, tell me I looked fine, but that just pissed me off more. Then he started getting mad at me for acting like such a lunatic. And I couldn't take it any more. I freaked out and screamed and threw my daily planner against the wall. Then I smashed my fist into the door. "You're fucking nuts," he said, and walked out of the room, slamming the door behind him. I threw myself on the bed for a minute then decided to chase after him. He had already turned around to come back, but I kept walking outside and he followed. I tried to calmly explain why I was so upset, but it turned into me yelling at him in the middle of the street for not walking with me and for inviting Jeff and for getting drunk on the plane. Thank God, Nick didn't try to fight back. He just listened, then gave me a hug and let me cry. Of course as soon as I calmed down I started feeling like a complete psycho loser, wondering how the hell I let myself get that upset. I suppose with everything going on in my life it was only a matter of time before I snapped. I just felt bad that Nick had to be the one I snapped on. But at least I had real tears for the "tearful, leaning on Nick" shots Donald had requested.

After all that, the appointment with Dr. Mauro was fairly anticlimactic. The biopsy didn't hurt me at all, but Nick was pretty freaked out by it. In a way I was glad. Once he saw me in the whole cancer context, he might be a little more patient with me, cut me some slack, let the fist slamming slide. He was really great, actually, asking good questions and taking notes as Dr. Mauro spoke. Dr. Mauro told us that even though I'd had a remarkable response in the first three months and it was likely that response would increase this time (again, we wouldn't get the results for a few weeks), I shouldn't discount bone marrow transplant as a viable option for the future. Doctors still doubted that Gleevec was a long-term answer to CML. Fortunately, the whole theory that you had to do a bone marrow transplant within 18 months of diagnosis to have good results was no longer common thinking. I could stay on the Gleevec until it stopped working and if I needed a transplant in 10 years, I could still do it then. The current thinking was that Gleevec could buy patients time, give them five, ten healthy years before having to have a transplant. In the meantime, transplant technology would improve and the risk involved would become less and less. In other words, the longer we put off transplant, the more efficient and safer the procedure would become. But I probably couldn't put it off forever.

Since I had pretty much stopped thinking about the transplant after finding out that only four percent of my cells had leukemia, this news was shocking to me. And it made me think about having babies again. If I were definitely going to have a transplant at some point, I would definitely be losing my fertility. But I still hadn't given up hope that I might be able to have my own kids someday. I asked Dr. Mauro what he thought about that. At that point two babies had been born to mothers on Gleevec. Both babies were fine, but one of the mothers had died shortly after giving birth. To be fair, she was in blast crisis, the most dangerous, life-threatening phase of CML, before she started taking the drug, but still, those odds didn't exactly make motherhood enticing. Dr. Mauro said that by the time I was ready to have kids, there would likely be some more data out there. There would be options, he said. We decided to put the whole having kids thing back on the back burner.

We left the hospital completely drained. Nick said it was really hard for him to see me in that setting, to realize that I was a real patient. It's easy to forget what we're dealing with when we're back in New York, living our fast-paced life, trying to squeeze one more minute out of every day. But when you spend two hours talking cancer facts and figures with your oncologist and getting the marrow sucked out of your bones and you actually take a second to slow down, the reality comes back full force. It kind of puts all the other craziness into perspective, something I really needed to do more often. Unfortunately, there was still more torture to come. The next day we had to go all the way back out to the coast with John so he could get some shots of Nick and me walking hand in hand on the beach. We were exhausted, but went out there and pretended to have a good time for the camera. Then we came back, packed up and went to bed. We were heading home the next day, and we couldn't wait. We'd both had enough.

My fourth column was about the trip to Oregon with Nick. When I turned it in, Cindi called Alison, who had taken over editing the column, very concerned. "Does Erin really mean all of this? Are she and Nick OK?" she asked. He did come off pretty bad in the first draft, and I felt a little guilty for exposing all of his immaturity, but I meant every word of what I wrote. Cindi just worried that if I left everything the way it was, we might get angry letters from readers telling me to break up with Nick. For a second I thought maybe I *should* break up with him. Maybe I deserve someone a little more grown up, someone who didn't like the couch so much, someone who was passionate about more than fantasy football and sex. A college graduate perhaps. But then I remembered why I was with Nick in the first place—because he made me laugh, because he was my best friend, and because in spite of all of his flaws, I loved him. And in spite of all of mine, he loved me, even if sometimes he had a strange way of showing it. I toned the article down a little so he sounded less like an asshole, and less like a lush. And the only letters we got about Nick said how lucky I was to have him in my life. And I was. I just wouldn't invite him back to Oregon with me any time soon.

The rest of the summer came and went in a flash, as summers tend to do. I had several speaking engagements, which were stress-inducing but surprisingly really fun. In fact, talking about my experience in front of large groups was becoming my specialty. My first big speech was for the National Young Leaders Conference in Washington D.C.—I would be speaking to about 350 ambitious high school students for 30-45 minutes about becoming a leader and giving back to the community. For weeks I worked on my presentation, staying up late to tweak my points, practicing for my family and friends, trying on outfits that said both "cancer research advocate" and "cool, young *Glamour* writer." By the time the day of the speech rolled around, I was so nervous I could barely eat breakfast.

I took the Delta shuttle to D.C. and Ronnie, another *Glamour* photographer, met me at the airport. For the first time in a long time, I was thrilled to have a photographer there. It was nice to see a friendly face. My parents had asked if they could come hear me speak, but since this was my first time, I wanted to go it alone. I'd be less nervous knowing that they weren't sitting in the audience hanging on my every word, my mom crying when I talked about my diagnosis and my dad cringing every time I said "um" or "like." Surprisingly, the moment I got up on the podium, I felt fine. I felt great, actually. The kids laughed at all my jokes and clapped at all my success with the trial and seemed genuinely interested in my story. Afterward, a bunch of them came up to me to introduce themselves and take their picture with me. I was so relieved that I had done a good job for them. And for me. And I was so grateful for the opportunity to be there, to be inspiring young people to do good things with their lives.

Unfortunately, the emotional high didn't last. I was flying back to New York that afternoon and had hoped that Nick would meet me in the city and take me out to dinner to celebrate. He said he might, but he wasn't sure he could make it. I didn't want to push him on the issue, mostly because I wanted him to come to the conclusion on his own that he should be there for me. I called him on his cell phone as we were pulling into the gate, and coyly asked where he was, half assuming that he would be at my apartment, maybe with flowers in his hand. "On my way to the golf course with Scott," he said. I was heartbroken. Exhausted and heartbroken. I told him I couldn't believe he didn't come in and he said, "You didn't seem like you cared one way or the other." "Well, I did," I said and started crying. He said he would ditch Scott and come to the city now, but at that point it was too late. It would have been after 9 p.m. by the time he got there. Plus, I was glad that he was hanging out with Scott—it had been really hard for him to leave all his friends in Knoxville, and I really wanted him to have a life in New York outside of our relationship. But I still cried for two hours straight. I was over-tired and over-sensitive—two things I seemed to be a lot those days.

I called my mom and she cried too, saying if she had known that Nick wasn't going to meet me she and my father would have come in and taken me out to a nice dinner. She was so upset and felt so bad for me that I had had such a big day and no one to share it with me. I honestly don't think she ever forgave Nick for not being there. When I finally asked her to stop mentioning it to me months later, she said, "It's just that as a mother you don't want anyone to hurt your child and when some selfish asshole does and there's nothing you can do about it, you want to kill him." I loved her for being so protective, but she needed to get over it. I had.

A few weeks after the D.C. speech I was at songwriter and philanthropist Denise Rich's Southampton estate speaking to 400 super cool, super fancy people, including David Guest, Liza Minelli and Star Jones (who does, in fact, wear Payless shoes). Denise had lost her daughter Gabrielle to leukemia in 1996 and set up The G&P Foundation, a charity that helps fund research for new leukemia drugs, in her memory. Every summer Denise holds a swanky fundraiser where everyone gets dressed up and parties and bids on amazing auction items like a first-class cruise around the world (opening bid: $20,000). And they raise a ton of money. In the six years since the foundation started, Denise had raised over nine million dollars.

Despite the fact that most of the auction items went for more than Nick and I make in a year combined, we didn't feel out of place at all, thanks to *Glamour*. When I first found out I'd be speaking at the party—which had a cabaret theme—I met with girls from the *Glamour* fashion department. They had access to all the best dresses from all the best designers and said they could definitely help me find something to wear. Unfortunately, most of the clothes that designers lend to magazines are samples, meant to fit stick-thin models who wear them on the runway or in fashion shoots. Sadly, I was not built like those models. But this didn't stop the fashion girls. "You can *so* wear a sample size," they said as they held up all the "totally fabulous" dresses they had called in despite my telling them that I could so *not* wear a sample size. To clarify, a sample size is around a 4. I wear a size 10. And though I could fit into the occasional 8, a 4 was nowhere within my reach. And I was OK with that. I'm 5'10" and most days I liked the way I looked in clothes. But even the most body-confident woman would start feeling like a beached whale after trying on 25 dresses without being able to zip a single one.

Each day for about a week I'd go into the *Glamour* fashion closet with a handful of fashion editors and interns. "I can't believe it doesn't fit," they'd say after each failure. "You do *not* look like a size 10." Finally, they decided they'd put me through enough torture and took me to Saks to just buy me something in my own size. Fortunately for me, that something wound up being a $1700 Halston dress—to this day, my prized (and most expensive) possession. Nick was able to borrow a Helmut Lang tuxedo—not because he was a sample size, but because the men's fashion editor was crafty and somehow got them to lend it to us in Nick's size. *Glamour* also sent a hair and makeup guy to my parents' house to make us—well, mostly me—extra beautiful. When we stepped out of the limo at Denise's house, we felt like movie stars (then we saw actual movie stars and started feeling a little more like regular people dressed like movie stars).

My job that night was to remind people why they were donating money. Novartis, the drug company that makes Gleevec, was a big sponsor of the event and had asked me to come speak about my experience with the drug—the PR person for the company had seen my *Glamour* columns. Fortunately, I had gotten the results of my latest biopsy back the day before and was able to work them into my speech—great for effect. "When I was diagnosed, 98 percent of my cells showed leukemia," I said. "Now, after just six months on this groundbreaking drug, less than *one* percent of my cells show leukemia." Everyone clapped wildly and I smiled, desperately trying not to tip over in the Badgley Mischka stilettos I'd borrowed from the *Glamour* shoe closet—unlike my ass, my feet could be squeezed into a sample size (a 9). "I know that as far as cancer patients go, I am lucky," I began to wrap up. "People have flus that are worse than what I've been through. But I also realize that I wouldn't be so lucky if it weren't for people like you who give doctors the means to come up with these miracles. I am proof that every single dollar you donate can make a difference in someone's life, even save a life. Thank you so much for everything you do." I got a standing ovation. When I got back to my table, I started crying. I couldn't believe that I was up on that stage telling my story. I was a cancer patient and that sucked but I was also as a cancer advocate and that was pretty cool. It was such an incredible night—and I really did feel lucky.

When I was first diagnosed, a lot of people told me I was lucky and I didn't really get it. Wait a minute, I'd think. Isn't getting a potentially deadly disease at 23 the exact opposite of lucky? Lucky is when I'm running late for work and catch the subway just before the doors close, or when the last pair of jeans on the sale rack is my size. Lucky is not finding out you have cancer on a perfectly nice Tuesday afternoon. Of course I knew what they meant: that with Gleevec in the picture CML didn't have to look so bleak. I just wasn't convinced. But after being on the drug for six months and watching my cancer disappear, I realized I am lucky. And not just because of that little orange pill.

In September, we took a family trip to my Aunt Donna and Uncle Neil's house in Florida. They have a great place in one of those utopian golf communities where every house is perfectly landscaped and there are more golf carts on the streets than cars. We were all there—my parents, my aunt, my sisters, Ysrael, Nick. Even Meghan's new boyfriend, Dustin, came with us, which I suppose wasn't surprising since he was living with my parents at the time. Meghan met Dustin in Panama City on spring break. He had dropped out of college and was 24 years old, so technically he wasn't on spring break, he was just there to hang out. (This would have been my first red flag.) He had a serious Southern accent (this would have been my second), but they hit it off from the moment they met—at midnight in a bar called Sloppy Joe's or something like that. They spent the last two days of Meghan's break partying together and after saying a tearful goodbye, promised to see each other again. The very next weekend Dustin drove up to Knoxville. Within a month, they were planning their life together.

Meghan fell for Dustin the way she'd fallen for photography and flying, completely convincing the rest of us that this was *it* for her, that she'd marry him and they'd live happily ever after. And my dad encouraged her passion the same way he'd always done, by overindulging it. Before any of us could object, he had agreed with Meghan's great idea and offered Dustin a job in his company. Dustin would move to New York, live with my parents until he could find a new place, and eventually go back to school. Never mind that Meghan was still at Tennessee and would be for another two years. Dustin could be in New York and start a life and then she'd join him when she graduated. "I'm gonna marry him, ya know," she'd say when Melissa and I told her she was out of her mind to let this happen. I think part of the reason she was so into him was because she wanted to be into him. As the youngest sister, Meghan was always trying to keep up with Melissa and me, to act older, to be included. We were both settled down with guys we loved and she wanted to be too. Never mind that he wasn't right for her. The plan was so twisted that even recalling it now makes me cringe. I just couldn't believe my parents would actually allow this. But they did. Meghan sent her boyfriend to New York, where he knew no one, to live with her parents while she stayed in Knoxville partying with her friends.

Fortunately, Nick had moved out by this point and gotten his own apartment in Huntington, but he was still working for my dad. Having Dustin do exactly what he had done made it seem trivial. Nick and I had been together for over two years when he moved up to New York. We were serious. Erin serious, not Meghan serious. And Nick had a lot of experience in telemarketing and sales, which is what he was hired to do for my father. It made sense. Dustin and Meghan had been together six months—all of it long distance—and Dustin had been working for his city's water utility. Not exactly the right training for my dad's business. They whole thing made my parents seem crazy, like they were running a halfway house for college dropouts. To be fair, Dustin was nice and thoughtful and he really loved Meghan. And he was way better than her last boyfriend (we never met the guy, but we later found out that the reason she broke up with him was because he was fired from his job at Corky's Barbecue Pit for showing up drunk). Still, the whole thing was ridiculous. Especially since we all knew it wouldn't last.

But at the same time, we were glad she had someone. After finding out that she was my bone marrow match, Meghan got pretty depressed. She wasn't just thinking about how great it would be to save my life, she was thinking about how horrible it would be if she gave me her marrow and then I died. Sure she had the opportunity to be the hero, but she also had the opportunity to let everyone down in a major way. Of course no one thought that way other than her, but I could see how she might be depressed by the whole thing. It was also hard for her to be down in Knoxville all by herself while the rest of us were up in New York going through everything together. Being removed from the drama can be good, but sometimes it can make you feel like an outsider, like you're uninformed, like people aren't always telling you the truth. Every time I'd talk to her she'd ask me how I was doing and if I answered with a "fine" instead of an enthusiastic "great," she'd say, "Why, what's wrong? Just tell me, Erin."

She started drinking more and sleeping more and eating more and going to class less. She gained a lot of weight and became even more sedentary and unhealthy than she already was. She said she would be sad and not even know why and then she'd think about me and just start crying. If teachers were mean to her, she'd start crying. If another driver beeped at her, she'd start crying, if she couldn't find anything to wear, she'd start crying. I knew the feeling all too well. When I talked to her I tried to tell her that I was perfectly fine—and I was—but she still worried. She felt like she had this big secret plaguing her and even though she had good friends to talk to, she still felt alone. Of course sending her new boyfriend to New York wasn't going to help, but she was in love and she had made up her mind.

As my luck would have it, the trip to Florida fell right in the middle of an injection cycle. At first I was really pissed that I'd have to stab myself with needles on my vacation—and that I wouldn't be able to sit on the patio drinking wine and getting sentimental with my sisters (I *could* do this without the wine but it wouldn't be quite the same). But then Melissa found out she wouldn't be drinking either. "Guess what," she said when she called me at work the day we were leaving. "I think I'm pregnant!" She blurted it out before I even had a chance to guess what. She hadn't taken a test yet, but she was three days late for her period and she just knew. She and Ysrael weren't trying—they were supposed to be waiting until they had been married a little longer and had a house and more money—but they weren't *not* trying either. Being Melissa, and loving attention, she decided to wait until we got to Florida to take a pregnancy test so we could all be there to watch. So, the next morning just as we were all waking up, she busted out of the bathroom holding a little white wand in her hand screaming, "I'm pregnant! I'm pregnant!" Dustin was the first person to hear.

From the moment the blue line appeared, Melissa was sure she was dying of every pregnancy problem in the book. She couldn't lift the "really heavy" dishes from dinner or exercise with me or stand the smell of chicken. She was completely nauseated and too tired to do anything more strenuous than walking to the pool and lying down. She didn't even golf. I'm not saying she was making it up—though I know my sister has a very low tolerance for pain and a very high one for attention—but my mom and I agreed that if she'd been the one to get cancer, she wouldn't have even made it past the diagnosis.

Still, she was overjoyed. All of us were. Even my dad, who had been warning Melissa not to "do anything stupid" and get pregnant before she was more financially stable, was giddy with excitement. For the rest of the trip, it was all we could talk about. We'd wonder whether it was a boy or girl, and who it was going to look like and what they should name it. "Now you guys have to get married and have a baby soon so our baby can have a cousin," Melissa said to Nick and me one night on the porch. "I don't think so," I said, laughing. Actually, Nick and I had been discussing that very thing earlier in the day. There was still no news on the fertility front, and we weren't quite ready to get married yet (especially after the last few months), but when we saw Melissa and Ysrael get so excited, we couldn't help but wonder if we'd ever get that chance. We had no idea what was going to happen, so we just clung to the hope that someday it might be possible, and we turned our focus back to Melissa. She was getting what she'd always wanted and we were so happy for her. And for us. It had been a tough year and we were all ready for some good news.

8 Here we go again

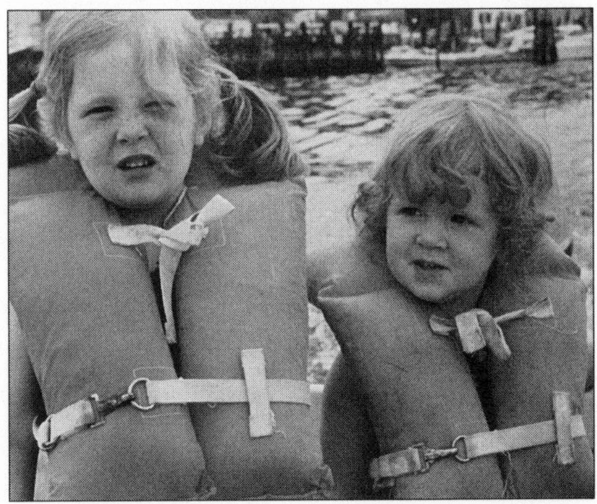

Melissa and me in our life-preservers on our dad's boat

FRIDAY, NOVEMBER 15, 2002 MARKED MY YEAR anniversary with cancer. My cancerversary if you will. It was a strange day—I wasn't sure if I should celebrate that I was still alive or be sad that I'd had cancer for a whole year and still wasn't cured (or in molecular remission). Really, I couldn't believe how fast it had gone. The first few days and weeks of my diagnosis were endless, like time was standing still, but since then my life with cancer had been flying by. The past twelve months were a blur of needles and pills and blood tests and weigh-ins—and, to be fair, plenty of normal life too. I briefly considered making Nick take me out to a fancy dinner so we could get deep and talk about how crazy it was that this time last year we were so freaked out and look at me now, but by noon I was over it. He picked up takeout sushi and we ate it on my bed while watching *The Breakfast Club* on TBS (not quite the same without the curses).

The day before Thanksgiving, Nick and I headed to Flint, making good on our rain check from the year before. I was glad we'd be spending some time with his family. I really liked them and wanted to get to know them better. Nick wasn't as close with his family as I was with mine, but he loved them and they loved him—and since someday they'd probably be my family, I wanted them to love me too. Plus, I was more than happy to escape the Zammett chaos, which only intensified over the holidays. It would start with my mom. Without fail, every time my sisters and I were home together, she'd find some totally mindless project that just *had* to be done, like cleaning out the barn or the basement or our closets. "OK, girls," she'd say, "I want you all to go through your old boxes of clothes and school stuff and decide what you want to keep. Whatever you don't want we're throwing out or giving to the Salvation Army." She'd start cheerfully—"C'mon, it'll be fun"—but if we slacked off at all, she'd change her tune: "No one is going anywhere until these goddamned boxes are out of my house!"

Meanwhile, the phone would be ringing off the hook. And though my parents had two portable phones, neither one could ever be found in time to get the call. "Is anybody gonna answer the freakin' phone?" we'd all scream in unison. Then, finally, one of us would step up, make a dash for the receiver, pounce on the speakerphone button and say "Hello" all breathless and annoyed. And despite the fact that my mom was always coyly saying, "Well, it's not going to be for me," it always was for her. Or for Meghan, who often got a bye on whatever annoying thing we were doing because she was either sleeping till noon after getting in so late the night before or getting ready to go out again that night. My parents didn't condone it, of course. In fact, half of the drama was my dad yelling at my mom for letting Meghan sleep—and then my mom screaming up to Meghan to get her little ass out of bed. "You *guys*," Meghan would say when Melissa and I complained about the inequity of the whole thing.

"I go to school so far away and I never get to see any of my friends." Poor girl. At least this year she'd have Dustin around to keep her from closing down the bars every night.

I also wouldn't miss my dad's inevitable flip-out over something stupid like my mom refusing to run a yellow light on the way to Aunt Donna's or someone eating his pumpernickel bagel or Melissa leaving her car window open when the weatherman had predicted rain (it didn't matter if it rained or not—even an averted disaster was a disaster). My father was less of a Grinch at Thanksgiving than he was at Christmas, but he'd still be wound very tight. And he'd be working on an elaborate, stress-inducing home improvement project of his own, like building a wall or tearing one down. That had sort of become his thing. The day after September 11, he decided that he was going to re-landscape our backyard with a short stone wall separating the patio from the back lawn. He and Ysrael (and Nick, when he'd make the mistake of stopping by to say hello) spent weeks ripping out bushes and tearing up roots and seeding grass and then laid every piece of Pennsylvania fieldstone themselves. It really looked beautiful, but it didn't last. A few days after I was diagnosed, my dad decided that the wall needed to be tweaked a bit and took every piece down and started again. No one could tell the difference of course, but redoing it gave him something to keep his mind off me.

My dad never stopped. Neither did my mom, for that matter. They were a good team in that way. They worked all week and they worked all weekend—even over the holidays. And they pretty much expected the same of my sisters and me who "didn't know how good we had it." Their house was cozy and homey and fun, but it was not relaxing at all. And sometimes I needed to relax.

Naturally, our trip to Michigan fell during an injection cycle. Every time I traveled or had anything important to do, I was on my chemo. It became a running joke—albeit not a very funny one. It wasn't easy to travel with a bunch of pre-filled, must-be-refrigerated syringes. I'd pack them in a little insulated lunch bag with an ice pack that invariably melted all over something that wasn't supposed to get wet. And by the time I got where I was going, the shots would either be lukewarm or ice cold, and I'd be convinced they were going to kill me. Surprisingly, though, for as many times as I flew with my needles, I was never once questioned at security. They'd always make me toss my eyebrow tweezers and take off my suspicious-looking sneakers, but somehow, no one ever noticed that I had a dozen hypodermic needles in my carry-on. Secretly, I wished someone would stop me, give me the third degree, try to make me leave them behind. Dr. Cathcart had given me a letter stating why I had to have them with me and I was ready to whip it out at a moment's notice. It would have been so satisfying, like getting carded right after your 21st birthday. But it never happened.

This time I was actually glad to have the shots with me—Nick's mom, Debbie, is a nurse and I was hoping to get her opinion on my injection technique. I'd been doing the shots for almost a year, but I still wasn't convinced that I was very good at it. Some days it went smoothly, didn't hurt at all, but others, it stung like a bitch. Sometimes I'd stab too hard and the needle would pop out a little, or it would catch in a weird way when I unpinched my skin. When Nick was with me, he'd immediately take the used needle from my hand for fear that I would start talking and gesturing with it and accidentally puncture myself, or worse, him. Neither of us thought I was the model injection giver, in part because I usually had one eye on the TV and my "hazardous waste" bucket was actually just an old milk carton that I kept in the corner of my room next to my hair dryer. A refresher course was all I needed—and maybe a lecture about taking the whole thing a little more seriously. Debbie watched me do the shot the first night we got there and said I did everything perfectly. Oh, well.

While we were in Flint, we saw movies and watched TV and looked at old picture albums. Nick showed me around the city—kind of scary—and Debbie and I went for walks around their neighborhood—also kind of scary—and we just hung out. We visited with Nick's grandparents, and when I saw all the letters he had written them hanging on their bulletin board I wanted to give him a big hug right there. As cool as he played it with his family, he was a really good, really sweet kid and I loved that.

In Nick's parents' house there was no work to be done. There was no yelling. There were no elaborate, boisterous dinners where getting a word in was like trying to jump into a game of double Dutch. The phone hardly rang. It was simple and easy and surprisingly fun. Debbie and I even had time to bond, which was great. We talked a lot about Nick, of course, mostly comparing notes on how he'd changed. She couldn't believe that he ate sushi and read books and ironed for me. I couldn't believe that he had gotten into as many fights as he once had—or that he'd taken ballet (it was only once and his dad made him do it for basketball but I'd still have to make fun of him for it). And neither of us could believe he liked rap music as much as he did.

We also talked about Debbie. She told me how she used to want to be a dancer and how she and Nick's dad fell in love right after high school and how when Nick and his sister, Michelle, were younger she worked Bingo and cleaned doctors' offices to make sure they had everything they wanted. She was really a great woman and I felt so comfortable around her. I knew that I would be lucky to have her as a mother-in-law someday. And except for the fact that no one at their Thanksgiving table had seconds—or thirds or fourths for that matter—I felt right at home.

Of course, the very next weekend I went to Huntington for a big dinner to get my fill of crazy—as nuts as my parents' house was, I couldn't stay away.

Melissa wasn't even three months pregnant yet, but she was already in serious maternity clothes, shuffling around with one hand on her belly and one hand on her lower back like she might go into labor any minute. She was also really sick, throwing up at least twice a day, napping all the time and leaving my parents' dinner table (where she and Ysrael ate most of their meals to avoid cooking and/or paying for groceries) in a combination of disgust and exhaustion. You'd think she was dying, not having a baby. She'd had a mysterious rash all over her body for almost a year and the pregnancy made it worse, so not only was she complaining about being nauseated all the time, she was scratching the shit out of herself. I did feel bad for her, but it definitely seemed like she was being overly dramatic—and like she was stealing some of my sympathy. Though everyone knew I was doing fine, I could still play the cancer card when I wanted to get out of doing dishes or emptying three tons of groceries from my mom's car. But now Melissa could play the pregnancy card, and most days that trumped the cancer card. And I suppose it should have.

At that point, I was still feeling really good on the Gleevec and I had pretty much learned to suck up the suckiness of the chemo shots. Even when I wasn't 100 percent, I rarely mentioned it to my doctors. I had begun to realize that sometimes a headache was just a headache and a couple of Advil would do the trick. And that there wasn't always going to be a profound explanation for every crick in my neck. Really, I just felt bad complaining. As far as cancer patients went, I knew I had it pretty damned good. My hair was still on my head, my body was still functioning fine and for better or worse, my life was still pretty normal. I had met enough people who weren't nearly as lucky as I had been, and if they weren't moaning and groaning, then I had no right to be either.

Three of those people were the women from the original *Glamour* story about Gleevec. When I was first diagnosed, some of my coworkers thought I should get in touch with them, find out what it was like to have CML, what to expect. I thought that was a terrible idea. Their experiences were totally different from mine—one quote in the article read, "I hurt so bad, I honestly didn't care if I died." Did I really need to talk to women who had been wasting away from a disease I just found out I had? I was also wary of the whole support group thing. I didn't want to sit around and trade depressing stories and feel bad for myself. I didn't want to be officially initiated into the sick club. But now that I had some distance from my diagnosis—and I knew I wasn't in danger of dying tomorrow—I thought meeting them was a good idea. So did my editor-in-chief, who wanted me to write about it in my next column. I called the women and introduced myself. A few weeks later *Glamour* flew them all to New York City for a little CML reunion.

The women arrived on a Friday afternoon. My stomach did flip-flops as I waited at my desk for them to call from the security desk in the lobby. I wasn't sure what to expect. Deep down, I feared they might resent me since they had all been so sick and had to fight so hard just to be let into the original Gleevec trials. All I did was show up feeling fine and I got the drug. But there was no negativity. In fact, they couldn't have been more supportive or more inspiring. After giving them a tour of the *Glamour* offices—and letting them pick out some makeup from the beauty closet—the four of us (plus Ronnie, the photographer) went out to a really nice, really expensive dinner on *Glamour*. We all ordered martinis and ate great food and talked nonstop about doctors and doses and side effects and surviving. If you were to overhear the conversation without seeing us, you might think we were a group of old ladies. But I didn't care. It was so refreshing to be with people who completely understood everything I was going through—even if it was as minor as "You know that gurgly empty pit feeling you get in your stomach after taking the pills? Doesn't that suck?"

There was only one thing that came out of the meeting that wasn't so encouraging. Though all three women had been doing exceptionally well on the Gleevec, one of them had decided to stop taking the pills three months earlier. She had been experiencing more side effects than most—she said the muscle cramping and fatigue kept her from doing the things she loved—and she had been in remission for a while and wanted to see if it would hold without the drug. So, against her doctor's wishes, she stopped treatment, hoping she could put the whole CML thing behind her. For the first month, everything was fine. But by our dinner, the amount of leukemia in her cells—which had been zero—was up to 28 percent. She needed to go back on the drug immediately. Even though I thought she was crazy for doing what she did, it was a sad reminder: No matter how healthy and normal I felt, I wasn't. My life literally depended on a drug. And considering that I'd spent my whole life taking care of myself to avoid that very thing, it was totally depressing.

Christmas was nice except that Dustin was there with my family and Nick wasn't, which made no sense at all. Melissa and I were actually kind of pissed that Meghan had invited Dustin to stay. It was OK that he'd be at the house for Christmas Eve, since half the town would be there for our annual party, but Christmas morning was a big deal in our family—it was one of the few times during the holidays when it was just us. The year before I was actually annoyed that *Ysrael* was there—and he was about to be married to Melissa. I couldn't help it. Sometimes I just wanted my family to myself. Growing up I always had to share their attention with whatever dinner guest or houseguest or neighbor was hanging around. And with other people there all the time, I was always trying to "be on my best behavior." I didn't want to have to do that at Christmas. But it was more than that. We all knew Meghan wasn't going to stay with Dustin forever (at that point, I think even she knew it) and now all of our Christmas '02 photos—and memories—would include "the dude from Alabama that Meghan used to think she was going to marry." Poor guy.

We skipped Aunt Donna and Uncle Neil's that year (lately they had been having Thanksgiving dinner *and* Christmas dinner) and instead, we had dinner at my parents' house with my mom's parents and sisters, who we didn't get to see as much. My Aunt Missy and Uncle Carl (who live in Massachusetts) and their three kids don't often come down for the holidays. They're all intense skiers—especially my uncle who can't bear to miss a day, even Christmas Day, on the slopes—so they usually spend Christmas at their ski house in Vermont. We used to go up there for a few days over Christmas break, but after the knee incident of '94, my dad refused. My Aunt Judy, who also lives in Massachusetts, would go to Vermont too, but this year, we begged and begged and they gave in and came to our house.

I always loved having my mom's family around. When we were younger, we spent almost all of our vacations with them, so my cousins, Erik, Mark and Kristen, were like siblings to us. We'd all stay up late playing games and talking and making fun of each other. My aunts were wonderful too, and always up for anything, especially drinking wine. And unlike everyone else in my family, they liked to exercise, even when it was cold outside. Only problem was, they both traveled with their dogs. Aunt Missy had a big, old golden retriever named Rossignol (after the skis) who shed so much you could have knit a sweater just from the dog hair in her car. And my Aunt Judy had an even bigger golden named Michael, who galloped around like a spooked horse but thought he was a lap dog at the same time. He was originally supposed to be a seeing-eye dog, but he got cut from the program when they discovered he had cataracts. I don't mind dogs, but at my parents' house, they sort of take over, like gremlins who eat after midnight. Especially that Christmas.

My parents had a golden retriever, too. Cassidy, who I had named during my Grateful Dead phase, was normally quite good but had a serious case of hyperactivity (she would play fetch until she almost passed out). This intensified around other dogs. Meghan also had a dog, a black mutt named Capone, who she and her three housemates at Tennessee had adopted together. Somehow, despite having four mommies—one of whom lived in Tennessee—Capone always wound up coming to our house with Meghan for the holidays. Fortunately, he was kind of like Eeyore and mostly stayed upstairs moping around by himself. ("He's probably overdosing on pills right now, Meg," Melissa and I would say to her when she couldn't find him.) Then there was my grandparents' little lhasa poo, Max, who humped all of the bigger dogs and when he couldn't find them, just walked around humping the air. Having five dogs in the house in addition to 15 gregarious, not-petite people wasn't easy. It didn't help that Uncle Carl had brought a laser pointer that he flashed around the kitchen so all five dogs would go nuts trying to chase it. "Cassie's going to have a goddamned heart attack, Carl," my mom yelled from the living room about a hundred times—when she wasn't busy screaming at Max to stop humping her toy soldiers.

Despite the fact that the house was literally a zoo, it was a perfect day. We watched Chevy Chase's *Christmas Vacation* about seven times (a holiday tradition), had a delicious and surprisingly peaceful dinner and played Piggy, my grandparents' dice rolling game where the winner takes all, usually 10 bucks. Even Melissa, who was still being plagued by her pregnancy, stayed up past nine and didn't complain too much. Everyone slept over and the next morning, we woke up to a massive snowstorm. We spent all day outside, building snowmen and snow forts and snow angels (and helping my dad shovel). I was so bummed that Nick was missing all the fun. He really was part of our family and it just didn't feel right without him there. I wanted him, not

Dustin, to have a dopey Santa hat with his name glittered on it. I wanted him, not Dustin, to get the matching golfing-Santa pajamas. And I wanted it to be him playing tackle football in the snow with my cousins. I knew he wanted all of that too—possibly even the glittered hat. When we talked, he promised that next year he would stay. I told him that I loved him and I missed him and I didn't want to spend another holiday without him. I wanted him around. Always.

A few weeks into the New Year, the Ara-C trial ended—a surprisingly bittersweet milestone. Though at times it was annoying, I would really miss having the attention of so many doctors and nurses and researchers. I liked knowing that they were constantly monitoring my disease and tabulating my results and having meetings about my case. I liked being patient 007. Of course I'd still have checkups and tests and doctors looking out for me but it wouldn't be quite the same. For one, my blood tests would be a lot less frequent, as would my checkups. And I'd be having my bone marrow biopsied every six months. These were good things, things that would make my life easier, but I couldn't help being a little nervous. What if something in my blood changed overnight and we didn't detect it for weeks? Would we still be able to catch it in time?

I would also miss getting my bottles of Gleevec Fed-Exed to me in a big package from the government each month. Now Dr. Mauro would be writing me a plain old prescription for it and I'd be picking it up at the CVS pharmacy on 25th and 6th when I got my birth control and my deodorant. This concerned me a bit—these were cancer meds we were talking about. Wasn't the neighborhood drug store too ordinary? The bells and whistles of the trial made sense to me, they made me feel special and different and without them I was just a regular old cancer patient. And since there was nothing regular about having cancer, that made me a little sad.

Perhaps the worst part about the trial ending was that the

chemo *didn't* end. Because I still had a smidgen of leukemia showing up on the molecular level (.002 at my last trial biopsy), Dr. Mauro thought we should stick with the injections for a little while longer—I wasn't so normal yet after all. I had suspected he might suggest this, so I was prepared. "I've made it this long, what's a few more cycles?" I said, trying to sound positive. But deep down I was bummed. The light at the end of my tunnel just got farther away.

Fortunately, I'd still be going to Oregon. When Dr. Mauro said he would be happy to continue to be my main doctor and to see me for my biopsies even without the trial, I was thrilled. Though I knew that Sloan-Kettering was the best cancer hospital around—and I really liked Dr. Cathcart—I'd never felt all that comfortable there. It was always packed and hectic and not everyone who worked there was as kind as you'd expect. There was also something not quite right to me about hopping a cab from *Glamour* to race up to my cancer appointment and editing "How to Make a Sexy Summer Cocktail" while sitting in the waiting room, then rushing back to the office to make the magazine's weekly production meeting. It was one thing to have blood tests and checkups at Sloan (which I'd still be doing), but I didn't want my cancer to become just something I squeezed in between seemingly more important things on my to-do list. Traveling across the country to do my biopsies was an event for me. Being out there gave me a chance to remove myself from my "normal" life so that I could focus on my abnormal life, if only for a few hours. And now that the trial was over, I needed that even more.

Since I was no longer following the strict trial protocol, Dr. Mauro let me stop the shots for my birthday, the big 2-5. I had another big party at another billiards place—I like people to have something to do while they get drunk—but this time I had Nick ask everyone for $20 at the door. Karen Travers, the girl who had interviewed me for the *Nightline* story, was running the

Dublin Marathon for the Leukemia & Lymphoma Society in my honor. She and I had become friends and I wanted to help her out—she needed to raise $4000 for the Society in order to make the trip. I invited my friends and coworkers, put up some LLS posters, ordered a few hors d'oeuvre platters and we had a party. Melissa even came in for it and actually stayed for a whole hour. Then she went back to my apartment to "die."

Ronnie was there again but after he shot a few rolls I told him to just have a beer and relax. There was nothing that compelling about seeing a bunch of young people drinking, even if it was for a good cause. Plus, we already had dozens of rolls of film from all the other parties I'd had. Donald had even started calling me the Paris Hilton of cancer (this was long before the sex tape scandal, mind you). He said he didn't want to see any more pictures of me dressed in black with my hair blown out and a wine glass in my hand.

But that was pretty much my life at that point. I had joined Denise Rich's cancer foundation as a member of the board, I was writing personal essays for various organizations' newsletters and I was still working a ton with the Leukemia & Lymphoma Society. I was averaging about one speech and two big party appearances a month. I was loving it—and fortunately Nick was now happily coming with me to everything—but it didn't exactly make for page-turning prose. Clearly, it was time for my column to wind down. The trial was over, I was feeling good and pretty soon I'd be stopping the shots altogether and then there would be no drama left at all. Of course I wasn't cured—the happy ending I had hoped for—and no one knew what the future held for me, but for now, at least, it was time to wrap it up.

As with the trial, I ended my column with mixed emotions. I wouldn't really miss the photographers—I had gotten tired of wearing makeup to my doctor's appointments and constantly stressing about how fat or thin I was going to look in the magazine (still hadn't quite gotten that whole perspective thing). I would miss the writing, though. Documenting everything I did as a cancer patient made my cancer seem like a character I could control. Seeing it in the magazine made it less real somehow, like it wasn't really happening to me, like I was just a reporter going deep undercover as a cancer patient. And while I knew that sharing my story helped some other people, it helped me even more. It made me feel less alone, it was my outlet—and without it, I was afraid I might not be so fine. But my seventh column would be my last.

In February, Nick graduated from college. It had taken him six and a half years, but he finally did it. His parents came in for the weekend and we had a big party for him at my parents' house. I wasn't sure how much he learned in his time as a college student, but I had gotten over caring about that. I just wanted him to have a degree so he could take advantage of every career opportunity that came his way (because I knew he didn't want to work for my father for the rest of his life—and I didn't want him to either). I knew that he needed to be a college graduate to open doors in his life.

My parents felt the same way, even though my father, who had been the head of sales for a multi-million dollar technology company and owned two of his own successful companies, went to college for about five minutes. I was always proud of this somehow. He was a completely self-made man—and he was one of the smartest, most driven people I'd ever known. When my dad was a little boy, he would wade out into the Long Island sound with an old zinc bathtub floating next to him and search for clams with his feet. He'd pack them into the tub, paddle back into shore and sell them door-to-door for fifty cents a dozen. When he was a little older, he would wake up before dawn, ride his bike down to the Sound, row out with a mask and a spear gun and hunt for eels, which he'd then take down to the fish market and sell to the highest bidder. Nick didn't have quite the same drive, but I knew he wanted to have a successful career in sales and that eventually he'd realize that in order to do that, he'd have to work really hard. Graduating from college was the first step and though at the time it seemed like it was more important to me, I knew it was a big accomplishment for him.

A few weeks after Nick's big day, I was back out in Oregon with my mom for my last regular biopsy before switching to the six-month schedule. With no photographer and no trial diary to discuss, the appointment was completely relaxed. I even attempted to pass off my cellulite as a side effect. "So," I said a little sheepishly, "I've been noticing an increase in the number of dimples on my butt—is it possible that the Gleevec is causing that?" "Um," Dr. Mauro said, searching for an answer while trying not to laugh. "I really don't think so." Bummer.

Mark came in during the biopsy and tried out a few of his new songs—I had started really looking forward to his performances (and his head massages) and even had Dr. Mauro call for him if he didn't come down on his own. We had a good old time. Afterward, my mom and I asked Dr. Mauro about the future, what to plan for. Through no fault of his own, Dr. Mauro didn't have many answers. There just wasn't any data out there that spelled out anything concrete for CML patients. At that point I was still in complete cytogenetic remission and really close to achieving molecular remission. We would stick with the treatment that was working so well and continue to monitor my blood for any changes. My prognosis, at least for the time being, was really good. And though I desperately wanted to know what this disease had in store for me, good for now was good enough for me.

At their seven-month sonogram, Melissa and Ysrael decided to find out the sex of their baby. Ysrael couldn't wait any longer and Melissa was tired of listening to him beg. But rather than have the sonogram technician simply tell them in the exam room, they had her write it down on a piece of paper and put it in a sealed envelope. Melissa wanted to make an evening out of it. My cousin Doug was getting married a few days later so all the cousins were in town and, naturally, hanging out at my parents' house. It would be the perfect night to make the announcement. So after a big steak dinner, we all gathered in the living room and watched Melissa and Ysrael rip open the envelope. "It's a boy! It's a boy! It's a boy!" they shouted together. We all clapped and hugged and even shed a few tears—it had been a long, hard pregnancy for Melissa, and she was in the home stretch.

At that point, she was feeling much better, but her rash was still in full effect and she had developed a strange lump on the side of her neck. When it had shown up a year earlier, she thought it was a pulled muscle. She went to the chiropractor for an adjustment, it went away a few weeks later and she forgot about it. But now it was back. Her gynecologist told her it was probably a small infection or a benign cyst, nothing to worry about, but that they should biopsy it just to be sure. For a world-class hypochondriac, Melissa was surprisingly calm about the whole thing. We all were. It wasn't like there was anything wrong with the baby—the thing we had been worrying about for seven months—and pregnant women always had weird, hormonal things popping up. We filed the lump with swollen ankles and varicose veins. No big deal.

On April 15, 2003, Dr. Mauro called to tell me the results from my biopsy. They couldn't detect the leukemia anywhere, even when they cranked up the sensitivity on the test to the highest level possible. I was in complete molecular remission. The CML might still be there, but no one could find it. After I asked Dr. Mauro a few questions—"Are you sure it's not a mistake?" "Can I stop the shots now?" "So this is really good, right?"—I let myself feel triumphant for a little bit. My last column, titled "One year into my battle with leukemia, I'm winning," had just hit newsstands and it couldn't have been more fitting—I *was* winning. I rarely celebrated my good results (it seemed like doing so would just be tempting the cancer gods), but this time I figured what the hell. As far as cancer patients go, I couldn't be in better shape. I was healthy and life was good.

Unfortunately, my happiness didn't last. Three hours after I got the call that I was basically cancer-free, I got a call from Melissa. It was in the middle of *American Idol*, her favorite show, and it wasn't a commercial break so I had a feeling something was up.

"Is everything all right?" I asked.

"Not really," she said. "Er, I have Hodgkin's lymphoma."

"Oh my God, Melis. Are you serious?" I asked.

She was. Apparently, the lump on her neck wasn't a cyst after all. It was a cancerous lymph node. The biopsy had come back positive that morning and her doctor had been trying to get in touch with her all day. She finally caught up with her at my parents' house and just like that, we were back to square one.

Melissa and I stayed on the phone for a while. Because I had done so much with the Leukemia & Lymphoma Society, I had a working knowledge of the disease, so I started spouting off facts. First, and most important, I knew that it was one of the most curable forms of cancer—more than 80 percent. And of the two forms of lymphoma—non-Hodgkin's and Hodgkin's—Hodgkin's was by far the better one to have. It was easier to treat and had a much lower relapse rate. I also knew that Hodgkin's was treated with chemotherapy and radiation, and that while the side effects could be pretty bad, most patients were still able to go to work. What I didn't know is how the hell a pregnant person deals with cancer.

I told Melissa that I'd call Dr. Cathcart first thing in the morning to get a referral for a doctor at Sloan, and I'd call the LLS to see what they knew. I also told her about every lymphoma patient I had met, and how they were now running marathons and doing Iron Mans and living normal lives, completely cured. I told her she was going to be fine, but I also told her that it sucked and I couldn't believe it. When I was first diagnosed, I appreciated people telling me I'd be OK, but I also liked people to say, "Holy shit, I feel so bad for you, that's horrible." I tried to do both for Melissa.

When we hung up, I dropped to my knees. I muted Clay Aiken who had been singing in the background the whole time and I sat there for a second, completely bewildered. Then I grabbed the phone and called Dr. Mauro. His voicemail picked up. "Hi, Dr. Mauro," I started, trying to stay cheery. "You're not going to believe this, but my older sister Melissa just found out she has Hodgkin's lymphoma." As soon as I got to "sister" my voice did that quivery thing and it was all over. "She's 27 and 7 months pregnant," I managed to get out through sobs. "Call me back if you can. Thanks, Dr. Mauro," my voice trailed off.

For a second I thought maybe we were on some cruel version of *Candid Camera*. How could this be happening to my family? No one would believe it—two sisters, both in their 20s, both diagnosed with blood-related cancers within two years of each other—but it was all true.

Lightning had just struck for the second time.

9 What's wrong with this picture?

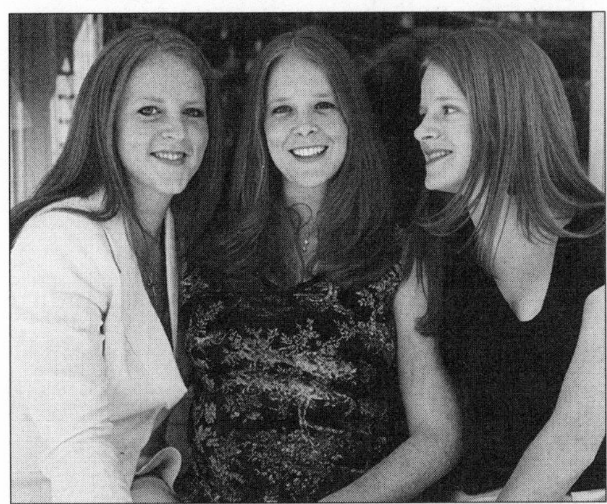

Meghan (left), Melissa (center) and me at Melissa's baby shower

WHEN I TOLD PEOPLE AT WORK THAT MELISSA HAD cancer now too, everyone assumed we must have grown up on a toxic waste dump. "Your parents are selling their house, right?" one of the more dramatic editors said. I suppose it was only natural to think that our cancers were caused by drinking water or power lines, that we must have grown up on Zammett Canal or a nuclear power plant or something, but neither of our diseases were linked to environmental factors. And they weren't hereditary either. Apparently, we just had bad luck. Really bad luck.

I had always said it was easier to be the person with cancer than to love someone with cancer and now I knew it was true. I felt so bad for Melissa it kept me up at night—all she ever wanted was to be a mother and now, just weeks before her dream came true, she had to deal with this. I worried about my parents too, maybe even more than Melissa. I suddenly realized how helpless they must have felt when they found out about me. And now they were going through those dreadful emotions all over again. Melissa told me that when they got off the phone with the doctor that first night, my dad just sat at the countertop with his head in his hands saying over and over again, "What the hell did we do wrong?"

But when you've been through it before there's only so much time you can spend getting upset. You know what to do and you just do it. And the one good thing about both of us having cancer was that I had connections. As pathetic as it sounds, with cancer treatment, as with many other things in life, it's all about who you know. And fortunately for Melissa, I knew people. The day after her diagnosis I got on the phone with everyone—doctors, nurses, social workers, patient advocates—and found out whatever I could about Hodgkin's lymphoma. Everyone was as shocked as we were to hear about the creepy coincidence, but they were eager to help. I was even able to get Melissa an appointment with the head of the lymphoma department at Sloan-Kettering less than 48 hours after her diagnosis. This was a huge triumph for me—if you can't use your cancer to hook your sister up, what good are you?

Once Melissa was diagnosed, it was as if my cancer disappeared. I didn't think about it as much or talk about it as much, and I felt healthier than ever. I wasn't doing the shots anymore, which helped, but it was more than that. In some ways, it seemed like I was passing the baton, like it was her turn around the track. So much of what we did and heard in those first few days was so familiar, and so many of the emotions we felt were exactly the same. But this time the stakes were much higher.

As it turned out, Melissa's new doctor's office was on the same floor as Dr. Cathcart's, just across the hall, in fact. I suppose it wasn't all that surprising considering we both had blood-related cancers, but still, it added to the "this is so fucked up" factor. Her appointment was on Good Friday, which somehow seemed appropriate, though I'm not sure exactly how. I took the day off and met Melissa and Ysrael and my mom up at Sloan. I had just been there two days earlier for my check-up, so it was a little weird—and kind of a relief—to be back and not be the patient. I showed them the best spot to get coffee and the fastest elevator to take to the fourth floor and introduced them to the receptionist, who I knew quite well since she used to work on the leukemia side.

My mom, Ysrael and I stayed in the waiting room while Melissa got her blood taken and had a chest X-ray (the only two tests they could do while she was pregnant). We talked about the same thing we'd been talking about since she'd been diagnosed—how we couldn't believe any of this was happening. After a few minutes of "who would have thoughts" and "not in a millions" I tried to steer the conversation to a more constructive place for Ysrael, who looked like he was either going to throw up or pass out or leave. His English had gotten much better since he'd been in the U.S., but he was still a little hard to figure out—I could understand what he was saying, but I never quite knew what he was thinking.

When Ysrael first moved to New York, every time he and Melissa had a fight (which was usually in front of the family since they were always around and Melissa kept nothing private) there was a part of me that feared he might just pack up and go back to Venezuela. He was dramatic like that. I knew he wasn't going to do that now, but I couldn't help but want to force him to see the bright side. I told him what a great hospital Sloan was and how all the doctors were so smart and how Melissa was in such good hands, but he just stared at me blankly. Nothing I could say would take away the fact that his wife, the mother of his unborn child, the whole reason he uprooted his life to move to America, was now a cancer patient. The situation sucked and we all knew it.

After about an hour of hanging in the waiting room, I took off. Meghan was coming into town for the Easter weekend and it was my job to pick her up from the airport and break the news. Even though we had all known about Melissa for two days, we decided to wait until Meghan got to New York to tell her. It would have been too painful for her to go through that over the phone twice. Plus, she was studying for finals again and my parents didn't want to disrupt whatever focus she might have. Of course since Dustin was living in Huntington (by that point he had moved out of my parents' house) and working for my father, *he* already knew, which seemed kind of unfair to me. But knowing how fragile Meghan was, I went along with the code of silence and so did he.

When I saw Meghan walking toward baggage claim with a huge smile on her face, I wanted to turn around and run. Now that my big sister had cancer, I couldn't imagine what it would be like to have *two* big sisters with cancer. It was so strange, and oddly powerful, to have that kind of information, to know something so big and bad, and to hold on to it for a few minutes longer than I should. I just knew that what I was about to say to her would change her life, take a little more of her innocence away, the same way it had when I told her about my cancer less than two years earlier, and that killed me. But I had to do it.

"So, you ready for the latest?" I finally said as we wheeled her bags to the car.

That was one of our family's favorite sayings, but it was usually followed by something relatively harmless like, "Melissa got fired for planning her wedding at work" or "You-know-who is drinking again." I figured using it in this case would help keep things light—at least until I said cancer, anyway.

"Oh, great, what now?" she asked.

"Um, you're not going to believe this but Melissa has Hodgkin's lymphoma," I continued. "But she's fine and the baby is fine and everything is fine." I looked up to gauge her reaction. She wasn't convinced.

"What does that mean?" she asked as the tears started welling up. "What's going to happen to her?"

As we got into the car, I told her everything I knew about Melissa's dianosis, which at that point wasn't much. Then I told her about all the lymphoma patients I'd met who had done so well with the treatment and were now cured and that Melissa would be just like them. And how Dr. Mauro (who, after receiving my frantic message, left me a voicemail at work, at my parents' house, at my apartment and on my cell) had been so reassuring when I talked to him. Meghan brought up worst-case scenario after worst-case scenario and I carefully fielded each one, telling her that Melissa was young and healthy and strong and that she was going to be OK.

Just as I was about out of bluffs, Melissa called us on my cell phone. Her appointment was over and she had answers. According to her X-rays, she had stage II Hodgkin's lymphoma, which wasn't the best but it wasn't the worst, either. Really, it meant that she had the disease in two parts of her body—in addition to the lump on her neck, she had a large mass in her chest that was pushing into her windpipe. This would explain why she hadn't wanted to do much exercise lately. I would try to make her go for walks with me sometimes, but after a few minutes she'd say she was out of breath and too tired to go on. We'd turn around and I'd call her a lazy, whiny pregnant lady. Whoops.

And the mysterious rash that had been plaguing her all that time? It was a *lymphoma* rash. This completely freaked us out. The summer before, when Melissa and I were out on my dad's boat filming the Leukemia & Lymphoma Society Jumbotron spot, she was scratching like crazy as usual and the woman who was taping us asked her what was wrong. Melissa explained that she had this awful rash that none of the specialists she had seen could diagnose—and that none of the hundred-dollar creams she'd been prescribed did a thing to stop it.

"I'm not trying to scare you," the woman said, "but my best friend had a rash like that and it turned out to be Hodgkin's lymphoma."

"Can you imagine?" Melissa said, laughing.

"Yeah," I chimed in, "I think me having leukemia pretty much rules out lymphoma for her."

And we thought that was the end of it.

The doctor figured Melissa had had the disease for about a year already, which meant she had it even before she got pregnant. Hodgkin's only affects a small percentage of the population, but it's fairly common in women in their 20s, so it wasn't unheard of for pregnant women to have the disease. In fact, Melissa's doctor had treated several mothers-to-be. The good news was, the baby would be fine. "Thank God," I said and repeated, "the baby will be fine" for Meghan, who was trying to read my face for clues. But Melissa needed to start treatment right away to shrink the mass in her chest—the way it was now would make breathing during childbirth nearly impossible. And the doctor wanted to avoid a caesarean section, as it would be too much of a shock to Melissa's already weakened system. So the plan was to give her a few rounds of Vinblastine—a type of chemotherapy that wouldn't harm the fetus—and then induce labor at 34 weeks. Melissa hated the idea of going so early, but was quickly learning to accept the fact that she had no choice in the matter.

"Then what Melis?" I asked as I carefully merged onto the packed Long Island Expressway. "When do you start real treatment?"

"Pretty much right away," she said.

Once the baby was out, she'd begin six months of aggressive chemotherapy followed by one month of radiation. She'd be getting ABVD, the classic Hodgkin's cocktail of drugs—unlike my disease, hers came with a very standard operating procedure. Of course she'd lose her hair and the chemo would make her tired and nauseated, but she should be cured. She'd even be able to have more children after being in remission for two years, a point Melissa emphasized: "Thank God, right?" she said. "I mean, can you imagine if I couldn't have any more kids? I'd rather just die." Melissa was definitely a little melodramatic, but being a mother was her biggest goal in life.

After I got all the facts, I handed the phone to Meghan so she could hear for herself how calm Melissa sounded—and so that I could focus on the rush-hour traffic. They talked for a few minutes, but when they hung up Meghan started crying again. "I just can't believe this," she said over and over. "I know, Meg," I said. "It completely sucks." And it did. But in typical Zammett fashion, we didn't get too deep or too emotional—there was no time: We had 60 women coming to the house the next morning for Melissa's baby shower. And Meghan and I were in charge of the decorations and the cake, which my mother had somehow forgotten to order.

Meghan couldn't believe that we were still having the shower, that we wouldn't have more time to talk about our sister and what it all meant. I couldn't either. I also couldn't think of anything worse than having half of the women in Huntington fawning all over me three days after I found out I had cancer. If it were up to me, I would have cancelled, given Melissa a few days to relax and let her diagnosis sink in. But my mom felt that the show had to go on as scheduled. Melissa might have cancer, but she was also having a baby—and that was worth celebrating. Melissa agreed: "What am I gonna sit around and be depressed?" she said when I asked her if she wanted me to make Mom cancel it. "I want presents!" I should have guessed. In fact, Melissa's only comment about the bad timing was that it was unfortunate we didn't know about her cancer *sooner*. "If people had known before they bought their presents, they'd probably be extra generous," she said, only half-joking.

So, within the six miles from the L.I.E. to Main Street in Huntington Village, Meghan and I switched from sad, tearful cancer mode to grin, bear it and shop mode. We only had an hour to get everything before the stores closed for the night. We went to the florist and the fruit stand and the party store, desperately hoping we wouldn't run into anyone who knew anything about Melissa—the only thing worse than feeling sorry for yourself is having other people feel sorry for you.

Everything went quite smoothly until we got to the bakery. First, we had to pick out the cake, which wasn't easy since almost all of them were shaped like Easter eggs or crosses. After about 20 minutes of debating—and briefly considering going with the whole Easter theme—we decided on the square carrot cake with velvety cream-cheese icing and little frosting carrots around the edges. It wasn't babyish or blue, but it had a certain maternal quality to it. Our next hurdle was deciding what it should say. "Congratulations Melissa" sounded weird in light of recent events, but we didn't want anything super cheesy or sappy either. We surveyed other people in the bakery, called my mom on her cell phone twice, and finally decided on "Showers of happiness for your bundle of joy." But our mission wasn't accomplished yet.

When the pimple-faced kid behind the counter grabbed a tube of icing, I knew we were trouble. "Don't they have special cake-writing people to do that," I whispered to Meghan as he started squeezing. This was one of the nicest, most expensive bakeries in Huntington and I couldn't believe my eyes. When he was finally finished, he tilted the cake toward us for approval. I started to cry. The word happiness was barely legible and the icing was hot pink. I knew it wasn't the time to be a perfectionist snob, but it also wasn't the time to give our cancer-ridden sister an ugly cake. In some ways, this was the most important cake we'd ever been asked to buy. It had to be perfect. But I really couldn't handle an altercation with this kid so I told him it was fine and gave him his money.

As we turned to walk out the door, my tears still streaming, Meghan grabbed my arm. "Give me that," she said, and took the cake from me. She headed back to the counter and said to the kid very sweetly, "Um, I'm sorry but this is a little messy. Do you think we can get a new cake and maybe get someone else to write on it? In icing that matches? It's for our sister and it's really special." Wow. I think that was the most proud I'd ever been of Meghan. She totally took control and managed to stay calm but still be forceful. Maybe there was hope for her after all. A few minutes later, we left with our new and improved cake in tow. We put it safely in the backseat, laughed at what a badass Meghan had been and headed to Rose Nail for last-minute manicures. We needed a little break before the chaos officially began.

As always, my mother was right. The shower turned out to be just what the doctor ordered. Melissa felt like a queen, everyone had a great time, and we were all able to think about something other than her cancer for while (like exactly how many Baby Boppies we were going to have to watch her open). We sat out on the deck and ate delicious food that my mom's friends had pitched in to prepare and drank mimosas and played silly shower games. Apparently there were some people who still didn't know about Melissa's diagnosis, but judging by everyone's enthusiasm for baby bingo, I'd guess it wasn't many.

Glamour even sent a photographer to document the festivities. It had only been a few days since the "final" installment of my column had hit newsstands, and already I was writing it again—as soon as I told my editor-in-chief about Melissa's diagnosis, she scheduled an update for the next issue. Melissa asked the photographer to take a bunch of extra shots so she could have them for her album—her holding up the outfit Grandma Ruth had given her, her with Joanna and the Diaper Genie, her with every burp cloth, booty and blanket she got. Melissa looked beautiful. Her hair was long and shiny and she was all baby. Of course we now knew that the reason she didn't gain much weight was because the cancer was eating away at her, but still, she looked great and wanted as many shots of herself that way as possible.

The next Monday, Melissa, my mom and a *Glamour* photographer went to the hospital for Melissa's first round of chemo. Fortunately, Sloan had a satellite cancer center on Long Island, so Melissa could get most of her treatment there and not have to go all the way into the city. She even got her own private chemo room, which was rare. (Melissa later found out the reason why: The nurses thought it would be too depressing for the other patients to see a pregnant person getting chemo.) Melissa was very cool about the whole needle-in-the-vein, chemo-pumping-through-her-body thing, which surprised us, considering her history of hypochondria. She'd actually been totally calm from the beginning. And in a way it made sense. Sometimes *thinking* you have something wrong with you is worse than *knowing* you have something wrong with you. You can drive yourself nuts with what-ifs and hypotheticals, but once you know it's true, you can take action, actually do something about it. And Melissa was all about getting things done.

"Tell Melissa what to do and she'll do it," my mother always said whenever she was comparing her three daughters, which fortunately she only did in respect to how we helped out around the house. Her favorite example was cleaning the kitchen. "Ask Melissa to do the dishes and she gets them done right away, no questions asked; ask Erin to do it, she'll put up a fight, make a lot of noise, but eventually get it done; Ask Meghan to do it and she'll 'yes' you to death, then 'totally forget' to pick up even one plate." In other words, to Melissa, cancer, like everything else in life, was very black and white—she got it, she'd beat it and she'd be done with it. No deep thinking, no second-guessing, no problem.

When the film from Melissa's first day of chemo came into the office, I could barely look at it. It was so bizarre to see her in her cute maternity clothes sitting in a big chair with an IV in her arm and a bag of liquid dangling above her head. Of course, being the exceptionally happy, roll-with-the-punches type of person that she is—and bad at acting natural when there's a camera around—Melissa was laughing in almost every frame.

Everyone used to tell me how well I handled having cancer, but I was quickly seeing that Melissa was by far the better patient. It did help that I had introduced her to the healing power of shopping. Within days of her diagnosis, we were at the mall spending money we didn't really have—and boy, did it feel good. On one of our early trips, Melissa decided to treat herself to a $300 pair of Chanel sunglasses and a Coach diaper bag. "If I'm going to be a bald mom, I'm at least going to be a stylish bald mom," she proclaimed as she threw down her credit card at almost every store we walked in to. Seeing how well the retail therapy was working on her, I decided to join in. I bought myself a pair of Seven jeans, a few shirts from Banana and a new lipstick. Afterward, we went to a fancy, waterside lunch (Melissa kept her Chanels on the whole time) and ordered virgin passion-fruit daiquiris. We ate chopped salads and gawked at the cute waiter and proudly re-lived each of our purchases. If it weren't for both of us having cancer, it would have been the perfect afternoon.

Melissa and I had always been close but we got even closer after I was diagnosed. Now that she had cancer too, we were like bosom buddies (sorry, Meg). If a day went by when we didn't talk at least three times, it was strange. But instead of depressing conversations about what was in store for her, we mostly gossiped about our family, bitched about work and planned exotic trips we knew we'd never take. If we did talk about cancer, we kept it to light, silly things, like how Charlie on *Party of Five* had lymphoma. And, as Melissa proudly recalled, "He lived. Or, wait, did he die?" We couldn't quite remember. We also talked about how totally bizarre it was that this time last year Melissa was being named Woman of The Year for the Leukemia & Lymphoma Society. "Just think about how much more money we could have raised if we had known!" she'd say. "We could be the freakin' poster family!" I'd agree. There was definitely a bit of novelty to the whole thing. And we were quite the hit at parties.

A few weeks after Melissa was diagnosed we were at a friend's barbecue and I overheard Melissa talking to a group of girls I'd never met, saying, "I have the curable kind, and she—Erin, wave!—doesn't. But I'm going to lose my hair and she won't." Jaws dropped all around. Unlike me, Melissa had no problem telling anyone and everyone she had cancer. I liked to be open about it too—obviously, I wrote a cancer column for a huge national magazine—but I tried to be more selective in whom I discussed it with. I tried to feel them out first, because sometimes they'd just get all quiet and sad and the last thing I wanted to do was make people uncomfortable.

Melissa got the chemo each week and continued on with her "normal" life. She didn't have any side effects so she was still able to go to work every day and at night help Ysrael finish the nursery, which at the point of her diagnosis had no paint, no furniture and no carpeting. I'd come home on the weekends to help her get prepared for her new life as both a mother and a cancer patient. This involved everything from framing Pooh pictures and buying diapers to trying on wigs.

Fortunately, Melissa had a little more time to get everything done. After her third round of Vinblastine, it appeared that she was responding well so her team of doctors—which now included a high-risk OB-GYN who Melissa saw twice a week for monitoring—decided to hold off on the induction until 36 weeks. Melissa was thrilled—if they took the baby at 34 weeks he would have had to stay in an incubator. At 36 weeks, assuming all went well, he could come home with her. After that news, she didn't worry about a thing. She was so closely watched in the weeks leading up to the birth that she didn't have to.

Everyone else wasn't quite as relaxed. My mom barely slept anymore and when she answered the phone, she'd immediately ask, "is everything OK?" no matter who was on the other line. Meghan was calling me from school every day to ask about Melissa and when I'd say everything was fine she'd accuse me of keeping something from her (I wonder why). And my dad was busy playing Erin Brockovich. Though all of our doctors had dismissed environmental factors, he wasn't giving up. He was reading books and searching the Internet and calling everyone he knew, desperate to come up with some explanation for why two of his girls had cancer. He wasn't alone, either. Nick made me promise not to drink the water at my parents' house (I had to remind him it was a little late for me), and Meghan set up an emergency appointment with every single doctor she could think of, even the dentist. Deep down, I also believed there had to be some reason all of this was happening, but there just wasn't time to deal with the whys right now.

On the night of May 20, 2003, Melissa gave birth—but it wasn't quite the one-two-three push that everyone had hoped for. Two days earlier she had been admitted to the hospital and given the induction drugs as planned. She had a few small contractions over the next day, but nothing major, so the doctor kept upping the drugs. Then, after two days of light labor and still no dilating, they had to go to Plan B: a caesarean section. My mom, who had been at the hospital with Melissa and Ysrael the whole time, called the house right before Melissa went in for surgery and 11 of us, including Melissa's best friend, Sherry, and my aunts and cousins from Massachusetts (who had come down for the festivities) piled into my parents' Suburban and hauled ass to the hospital—Nick was the designated driver. We got there just in time to see Melissa getting wheeled out of the operating room, with a beaming Ysrael by her side and her new baby, Andrew Rafael, in her arms. She picked the name Andrew so that she could call him Drew—because all Drews were hot, and *her* son would definitely be hot.

After a minute or two of letting us ooh and aah, the nurses carted Melissa off to recovery and Andrew off to the nursery. We followed the baby and watched through the glass as the nurses washed him and weighed him and measured him. He was 6 pounds, 8 ounces and 20 inches long—not bad considering he was a whole month early. We spent about two hours with our noses pressed against the glass, pointing out each perfect finger and each perfect toe. Then we headed home, huge smiles spread across our faces.

Melissa and Andrew came home from the hospital three days later. They went directly to my parents' house, where they and Ysrael lived for a few weeks so my mom could help with the baby while Melissa recovered from the C-section and prepared for the chemo. She was healing nicely and feeling pretty good considering what her body had been through over the past month. In fact, the only real pain she had was in her boobs. Since the chemo would essentially turn her breast milk into poison, Melissa wouldn't be able to breastfeed (this devastated her until she realized it meant she could drink wine again a lot sooner). To force her milk to dry up, she had to bind her chest by wearing two of my B-cup sports bras for about three days. Even when they're not full of milk, Melissa's boobs are DDs, so she was pretty much in agony. Still, she didn't complain. She felt like the luckiest person alive. She had everything she'd ever wanted and nothing—not even cancer—could take than away from her. Damn, she was good.

With Andrew around, we were all in heaven. You'd think

that having a baby right before starting major cancer treatment would be poor timing to say the least. But it couldn't have been more perfect. He was just so cute and cuddly and peaceful that we couldn't help but be happy. We fought over who got to feed him and hold him and change his little diapers. Even my dad was talking baby talk—mostly about how he was going to teach Andrew to fish and golf and root for the Mets. Andrew's arrival was bittersweet, though. Now that he was here, Melissa's life with cancer would officially begin.

10 Remission, hope and mojitos

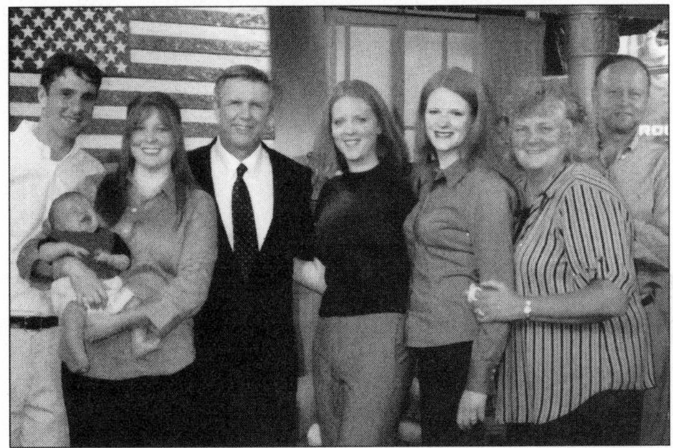

The whole family with Charlie Gibson after our Good Morning America *interview*

After enjoying motherhood for a whole week and a half, Melissa headed back to the hospital to do all the fun tests she couldn't do while she was pregnant—bone marrow biopsy, CAT scan, PET scan, etc. Two days after that, she and Meghan, who was home from school for the summer, went to her oncologist's office to get the results. Not surprisingly to any of us, they weren't very good. Apparently, the Vinblastine she had gotten during her pregnancy didn't work well at all. The lump in her chest was still there and bigger than ever. Even worse, she had failed her pulmonary function test (a lung capacity thing), which she needed to pass in order to take Bleomycin, the B in the ABVD regimen they had planned to start her on. So since she wouldn't respond to the V and couldn't handle the B in the ABVD, they scrapped that plan and instead decided to do something called Stanford Five, a newer, more intense form of treatment. At first, Melissa was fine with the change of plan, especially since Stanford Five only involved three months of chemo and one month of radiation, which was considerably shorter than the ABVD. But then Meghan asked about the long-term effects of the new drugs.

"The Stanford Five will 'render' me fucking infertile," Melissa said to me when she called in a panic from the car on her way home. Evidently, a potential side effect of nitrogen mustard—one of the five drugs in Stanford Five—is infertility. And we all knew Melissa wanted no part of that. In fact, before she left she told her doctor she'd like to go ahead with the ABVD even if now it would only be AD. There was no way she was losing her fertility. We all tried to talk some sense into her, but she wouldn't listen. I think she really believed that she'd rather die than not be able to have more kids. When Nick and I talked about it that night, he couldn't understand how crazy she was being—especially since I had taken my fertility news so well. "I'm so glad you don't act like that," he said. "Doesn't she realize that all that matters is that she gets better?" She didn't.

The next day, Melissa and Meghan headed back to the hospital, assuming that Melissa would get her way. But when they arrived at the chemo room, Melissa's doctor handed her a phone. The head oncologist from Sloan was on the line and she was not pleased. "If you continue with the ABVD you will most certainly relapse within a year and have to have a transplant," she said matter-of-factly. "Then you will *definitely* be infertile. I want you to go home and take a good look at the baby you already have. If you want to be around to watch him grow up, you've got to do the Stanford Five. It's just that simple." Melissa understood and actually respected the doctor for speaking so bluntly. I think I would have died if one of my doctors talked to me like that—I can handle the truth, but I need at least a spoonful of sugar to swallow it.

The doctor also told Melissa about a drug called Lupron that they were using to put female cancer patients into false menopause during treatment to protect their eggs. There was no proof that it would counter the effects of the nitrogen mustard, but it wouldn't hurt. That was all Melissa needed, a little glimmer of hope. She was sure the Lupron would work for her and that she'd be popping out another kid in no time. She hung up with the doctor, sat down in a chair and got her first round of drugs.

A week later, Melissa was completely bald—but it wasn't because of the chemo. Knowing that her hair was going to fall out soon anyway, she decided to go for the preemptive strike—get it all cut off and have a wig made from it. She had done her research and found Rodolfo Valentin, a famous hairdresser who had lost his mother to breast cancer. He made beautiful wigs—"hair prosthetics," he called them—and donated them to cancer patients. Melissa called him up and he agreed to make her one using her own hair as long as she donated the wig back to him when she was finished with treatment. It was a deal.

My mom, Meghan, Andrew and I all went with Melissa on the big day for moral support. We figured we'd be there for an hour or two, tops. It was more like five. Turns out, having a wig made is an intense production. There were fitting apparatuses and molds and markers and assistants running around frantic and, of course, the age-old hair question: bangs or no bangs. I suppose having your head shaved is much less depressing than letting your hair fall out strand by strand, but still, we all cringed as Rodolfo started buzzing Melissa's scalp. My mom, of course, took pictures. And cried. It was just so heartbreaking to watch Melissa be transformed from happy, healthy new mom to sad, bald cancer patient right before our eyes. But if anyone could pull off the hairless look it was Melissa. She had a beautifully symmetrical face, a perfectly round, dent-free skull and a lot of confidence. "It's a good thing I have such a pretty face," she said as we left Rodolfo's.

Rodolfo gave Melissa a temporary wig that she'd have to wear for a few weeks while his team sewed each strand of her hair into a new wig by hand. It looked really good, really real, but we all knew what was underneath: a bald head, the universal symbol for cancer. It was especially hard for my dad and Ysrael and Nick to see her. The guys in our family just didn't handle the realities of cancer as well as the women did, and the reality of Melissa's new hair was that it screamed, "I have cancer and I might die." The day after Melissa's bald debut, my father decided to knock down the wall between the foyer and the guest room and build a big formal dining room. Some people turn to God or to booze in times of despair; my father turns to his hammer and nails.

My dad is the quintessential do-it-yourself guy—and often escapes reality by building things. One of the many previous job titles he'd held was carpenter, so he's skilled and actually built most of our house himself. He used to have a woodshop in the basement and was constantly down there creating something. When my sisters and I were younger we'd be his assistants and if we were good he'd build us stuff like little airplanes that we spray-painted gold and step stools with our names carved into them so we could reach the sink to brush our teeth. I used to love to go down there and hammer with my dad and watch him use the blowtorch and press my hands against my ears when he turned on the table saw. Then one time I went down in my floor-length flannel nightgown to show him the high kick I had learned from Grandma Del in dancing school that day. With my hands firmly placed on my hips, I put all of my energy into kicking my leg up as hard as I could. Only I forgot to pull up my nightgown so when my leg hit the front of it, it became taught between my two legs and the momentum from my kick carried me right up into the air and backwards onto the cold, hard concrete. I survived, but it was a while before I went down to the basement again.

My dad is also interested in plumbing and electrical systems and when we were younger, he would often regale us with tales of his genius, like how when I was born—during the blizzard/blackout of 1978—he used boat batteries and taillights from a car to rig up an elaborate lighting system in the house, complete with on/off switches. He was always refiguring something or rewiring it or rebuilding it—all while running his company, which was conveniently located two and a half minutes from the house (and across the street from the boat). Keeping himself busy was the key to my father's sanity—especially lately. As long as he had something to build, he wouldn't have to think about how his beloved family was falling apart before his eyes.

For the next three months, Melissa had chemo once a week. She'd go to the hospital, get hooked up to a machine and sit there for anywhere from one to three hours depending on which drug she was getting. *People* and *US Weekly* became her new best friends and she'd often call me from the chemo chair to say things like, "Oh my God, did you hear that Ben Affleck and Jennifer Lopez are dating?" Duh. She and Ysrael had moved back into their apartment, and she was able to do all of Andrew's feedings and cook nice dinners (or at least go to my parents' and eat nice dinners) and have sex and drink wine. She tolerated the drugs remarkably well and only got sick twice—once because she scarfed down a bacon, egg and cheese sandwich too fast and once because her nurse screwed up and forgot to give her the infection-fighting drug she was supposed to get with her chemo. That one was pretty bad.

It was the day after she had gotten the nitrogen mustard, the one drug that knocked her down a bit, and when she woke up she was feeling exceptionally crappy. Ysrael noticed that she was burning up, so she took her temperature (all cancer patients are taught to be wary of fevers). It was 104. She called her doctor who told her to get to the hospital right away.

Of course the timing couldn't have been worse. My mother had just left town with a few of her girlfriends for a much-needed getaway and Meghan was back at school (she had to do a semester of summer school to make up some credits). Ysrael was going to stay home from work to take care of the baby, but that left only my dad to drive Melissa the half hour to the hospital.

At first, he was uncharacteristically calm, driving normally, asking about Andrew, making sure Melissa was comfortable. Then Melissa made the mistake of telling him exactly how high her temperature was. "What??!!" he yelped. "You could get brain damage if we don't get you there fast enough." And just like that, he turned into the maniac we all know and love, screeching around corners and running lights and blasting his horn at anyone who got in his way. By the time they made it to the hospital Melissa was screaming at him to relax, telling him that it was no big deal, that she would be fine. Despite the fact that he was never the patient, when it came to emergencies, my dad usually needed the most care.

The doctor at the hospital wanted to admit her, but that would have meant three days away from Andrew, so Melissa refused. She promised to take it really easy and the doctor relented, allowing her to get the antibiotic drip as an outpatient. My dad stayed with her all day while various fluids pumped through her body. By six o'clock, they were free to go home—Melissa was still feeling pretty bad, but her fever had broken and she was no longer at risk for major infection.

Since my mom was out of town—and Melissa and I didn't want her to have to come back like my dad suggested—I decided to take the next day off from work and head to Huntington to help out. I met Melissa and Andrew at my parents' house, where we were all going to spend the night. Nick came over too. Ysrael stayed at their apartment so he could get some sleep. I told Melissa that Nick and I would be able to handle all the nighttime feedings so she could just sleep and relax.

"C'mon, it'll be fun," I said to Nick when he looked at me like I was crazy. "We can pretend he's our baby." Nick didn't seem quite as excited as I was, but he helped me move Andrew's crib into the room with us.

At the midnight feeding, everything was fine. Andrew woke up, he took his bottle, I burped him and he went back to sleep. But after the 3 a.m. feeding, I couldn't get him to go back into his crib. I'd try to put him down every few minutes but he'd just start wailing again. After about 30 minutes of this routine, Nick said he couldn't take it any more, put on his clothes and went back to his apartment. Nice. At that point I gave up on the crib and decided to just put Andrew in bed with me—but that turned out to be even worse. He had stopped fussing but I was so afraid that he would fall out that I could barely breathe, let alone close my eyes. Fortunately, Melissa came into the room at 4 a.m. and said she was feeling better and she could take him back. I tried to put up a fight, but I was so tired and defeated that I just let her take him.

Luckily for the rest of us, that was the worst it ever got for Melissa. From then on, she really handled the chemo like a champ. This was a positive thing, of course, but sometimes I think she felt a little *too* good, considering she was still a cancer patient going through serious treatment. Melissa drank like a fish all summer. Once, she even showed up for chemo with a serious hangover. But if we tried to say anything to her, to get her to have *two* glasses of wine with dinner instead of *four*, she'd just get mad. She'd say it was her prerogative after carrying a baby for nine months (eight, I'd remind her) and that her diagnosis made her realize that life was short and that she needed to enjoy every day and for her that meant having as much damned wine as she pleased. To me, this was just blatant abuse of the cancer card—but it worked.

So did all that wine, apparently. In the beginning of August, Melissa had a PET scan to look for cancer activity and it came back negative. She was in remission. She still had a couple more weeks of chemo left and the month of radiation to do, but her cancer was gone. I was impressed, overjoyed, relieved—and a little jealous.

In September, we were back down in Florida drinking wine on Aunt Donna's porch and listening to my dad relive each shot he, Nick and Ysrael had taken on the golf course that day. He had a Rainman-like ability to recall in full detail not only every drive, chip and putt everyone in his foursome had made, but also which way the wind was blowing on a particular hole and how the hot dog tasted at the turn. "You should never come up short when you're puttin' for birdie," he said, lighting a cigar and taunting Nick about his choke on the 14th green. This was one of my father's favorite golf mantras and he used it on all of us, often. Of course if he were ever the one to come up short, this little chant would be accompanied by some four-letter words and, occasionally, a club smash. But my father rarely broke his own rules.

We had decided to head down to Florida after Melissa finished chemo. She had two weeks off before starting radiation and the airline was practically giving the tickets away so we figured what the hell. We could all use a little R and R (and G). It was the same players as the year before minus Dustin, who was no longer in the picture. After months of having doubts, Meghan had finally broken up with him right after Andrew was born. A few days after that, Dustin had quit his job with my dad and moved back to Alabama. We had seen that one coming for a long time, but for better or worse, Dustin had become a part of the family and knowing he was heartbroken broke our hearts. Meghan felt bad too, of course, but she also felt really good.

Since Christmas, Meghan had changed. She wasn't smoking anymore, she wasn't eating bad foods and she was exercising almost every day. By the time we were down in Florida, she had lost 30 pounds. At first we thought this lifestyle change was motivated by the fact that both of her sisters had cancer and she realized she'd better start taking care of herself. But as it turned out, it was because she was tired of coming home every holiday and listening to us tell her she needed to get healthy—she just wanted to shut us up, to prove to us that she could do it. I think it also had a little something to do with the fact that she knew she didn't want to be with Dustin, and if she was going to be single again she needed to whip her ass into shape. Whatever it took, I said. She looked amazing and for the first time in a long time she and I were getting along great—she actually wanted to take walks with me and do sit-ups with me and split dessert. Even at school she'd get up early (well, 10 a.m. as opposed to noon) and go to the gym and eat Lean Cuisines instead of Papa John's pizzas. I was so proud and so relieved. Finally, I wasn't the only in-shape sheep in the family.

We had a blast down at Aunt Donna and Uncle Neil's, playing golf and tennis every day, eating delicious dinners every night and watching Andrew roll over and splash around in the pool for the first time. And Melissa was feeling great, so, for once, nobody really talked about cancer. She was still bald, but we had all gotten used to it—after all the trouble she went through to get the wig made, she really didn't wear the thing very much. It was too damn hot. So when it was only family around, she'd skip the scarf or bandana and just wear nothing at all. At first it was weird to see her sitting across the table with less hair than Andrew, but like everything else, we just got used to it.

Melissa's head wasn't the only thing that was different, though. She'd also been getting quite round over the previous few months. Melissa had always been a big eater, but after she was diagnosed, she took the "you only live once" approach to every burger, bagel and bratwurst that crossed her path. She blamed her puffiness on the prednisone she had been taking (which, to be fair, did cause water retention and an increased appetite), but we all knew it had more to do with the thousands of calories she was chasing the pills with. Melissa had always been happy with her curvy figure and I loved that about her, but she was quickly exceeding curvy. By this point, she weighed more than she had weighed the day she gave birth to Andrew—*before* he came out. I tried to explain to her that someday soon she'd be done with the whole cancer thing and then she'd have the whole fat thing to deal with and that would suck, but she didn't care. She looked like the Pillsbury Doughboy and it didn't faze her in the least. I should have known. Melissa wasn't nearly as obsessed with her body as I was with mine and she never worried about what other people thought of her. Lucky bitch.

While we were in Florida, Nick and my dad talked a lot of business, as they tended to do whenever cigars and Sambuca were involved (Nick wasn't especially fond of either but enthusiastically partook in them to please my father). Because the data storage business was so high tech (read: boring), the rest of us would head inside and leave them on the porch with their stogies. In the two years that he'd been working for my dad, Nick had proven himself to be quite an asset. This was a good thing, of course, but it also created a bit of a conflict for Nick and me. At some point soon, we hoped, Nick would move into the city and get a job where his boss wasn't my father. He enjoyed working for him, and he had learned a lot, but we were both tired of having every aspect of our lives entangled with my parents.

My mom did the books for the company so she knew exactly how much money Nick made each month and what hours he put in. "Nick sure doesn't stay a minute past five, does he?" she'd say to me every once in a while. God, I hated that. Working for my dad also meant that Nick was on call 24/7 to do whatever my dad wanted him to do—help him clean the boat, drive Meghan to the airport, come over for steaks. These things weren't in the job description, but they were definitely part of the deal. Nick had absolutely no separation between his work and personal life, and he wasn't exactly itching to spend more time with my parents on the weekends. But that was the only time I got to see them, and I really looked forward to our big dinners together. I knew if we were ever going to get married and have a life together, Nick would have to leave my dad's company. We just had to figure out a way to break the news to the boss.

Back in New York a week later, Melissa got prepared for her radiation. The chemo had already gotten rid of the cancer, but as part of the Stanford Five protocol she needed to have radiation—it was an extra step to ensure that the cancer wouldn't come back. This "insurance policy," as some doctors called it, didn't come without a price, however. Radio waves—especially in the chest area where Melissa was getting them—could lead to a host of other problems, like breast cancer, lung cancer and even leukemia. Naturally this freaked us out, but we couldn't worry about it right now. One disease at a time.

Before Melissa could start the radiation, she had to get little freckle-like tattoos on her body so that the technician would know exactly where to line up the machine each day. They strapped her to a table and told her not to move a muscle. She lay like that for an hour while they poked her chest and sternum and stomach with needles full of ink. "It was pure torture," Melissa said when I met her and my mom for lunch afterward. Fortunately, that would be the hardest part of the radiation process. After that, all she'd have to do is go into a room and lie down on a table for about 20 minutes. *Unfortunately*, she had to do this part of her treatment at Sloan-Kettering, which meant she'd be traveling for about three hours just to get to those 20 minutes. And she had to do it five days a week for a whole month.

Melissa was pretty hardcore about the whole commuting thing. She was back at work part time at that point (she went back even before her maternity leave was up—as the breadwinner in the family, she had to), so she'd work half a day, then walk from her office to the train station, take a train to the city, then get on a crosstown subway, then switch to an uptown subway, then get out and walk three avenues to the hospital. After she got zapped, she'd turn around and do it all over again in reverse. As someone who refused to take the subway at all for the first three months of my diagnosis—and never once took it to Sloan—I was thoroughly impressed.

On Thursdays, Melissa would do her radiation late and spend the night at my apartment, then do early-morning radiation on Friday before heading to work. When she first came up with this plan, I figured we'd lay low on those nights, order in sushi or Mexican, watch *Friends* and *Will & Grace*, get a good night's sleep. But it never quite worked out that way. Despite the fact that the radiation gave Melissa a sore throat and a painful burn on her chest, she always wanted to go out afterward. She'd say it was her one night without her husband and her baby and she had to make the most of it. So we'd go to fancy restaurants and wind up eating too much and drinking too much and staying up well past midnight.

We'd have a great time, of course, but it wasn't exactly healthy living. Each week I'd tell Melissa that we had to be good, that I didn't want to overindulge or stay up too late, that I had to go to work the next day and so did she (God, I was boring). She'd agree to take it easy at first, but slowly she'd win me over to the dark side. "C'mon, Er," she'd say when she got to my apartment, "I just came from having radiation to cure my cancer that in the process will probably give me *more* cancer. I need a glass of wine."

I definitely learned more about cancer and life from Melissa than she could have ever learned from me—the most important lesson being to play the cancer card on *myself* every once in a while, to stop and say, "Hey, you have cancer, sleep late, have a cheeseburger, lighten up!" In some ways, getting cancer made me even more of a control freak. When I was first diagnosed, I did slow down a bit, but soon enough I was right back to my old habits. I still wanted to do and be everything I could despite the fact that I had this disease—to spite it, maybe. This was a good attitude to have, I think, but sometimes in the process of trying to be perfect, I forgot to just enjoy life. Melissa reminded me to do that. Those nights we had together became like our own personal support group and I cherished them—Friday morning hangover and all.

Meanwhile, I was writing my column regularly again (documenting Melissa's experience as well as my own) and giving a ton of speeches. Now more than ever, I felt compelled to share my story. When Melissa was first diagnosed, I was constantly talking about all the lymphoma patients I knew who had done so well, and that's when it really clicked: Cancer patients—and their families and friends—need to know that there are people out there just like them who are surviving, people who can inspire them and give them hope. I could do that with both of our stories.

Speaking about Melissa's experience wasn't quite as easy as speaking about my own. I had gotten so used to talking about my cancer that it didn't seem real anymore, but hers was so fresh. And saying the words out loud just reinforced how shitty the whole thing was. Every time I would get to the part of a speech when I mentioned her diagnosis, I choked up. It was one of those moments of pure reality where you realize exactly what's going on in your life—and how much that sucks. On the plus side, talking about Melissa's diagnosis was great for impact. "She was 27," I'd say, pausing, "and seven months pregnant." And the audience would gasp.

Our story was so unusual that we were even featured on

Good Morning America—Charlie Gibson interviewed Melissa, Meghan, Andrew and me live. This was totally nerve-wracking, especially for Melissa who tends to laugh a lot and stumble over her words when she's nervous. "I'm worried that when I describe the chemo I did while I was pregnant, I'm going to say that it didn't harm the *feces* instead of the fetus," she confessed in the car on the way to the studio. Fortunately for all of us, she didn't make that mistake. She did make a goof but it was a far less embarrassing one. When Charlie asked her what it was like to have the *Glamour* photographers follow her around, she told him she loved it. "It helps make the whole thing more dealable," she said. Of course dealable is not actually a word, which Melissa realized as soon as we finished the segment. "It should be a word," Charlie Gibson said to console her. "It makes sense to me." He was a very nice man.

If cancer were a competition—and really, everything in my family is—Melissa would definitely win. Within six months of her diagnosis, she had given birth to a healthy baby, completed chemo and radiation and achieved full remission. And she'd done it all without so much as a grumble. A few days after her last round of radiation, she threw a party to celebrate her success, something I wasn't very keen on at first. I was thrilled with her remission, but I was a bit wary about having a farewell-to-cancer fête so soon after her treatment ended. It just seemed too easy to me. Could this really be it for her? Could she have put cancer behind her so quickly? I wasn't so sure. But then I was always a little skeptical when it came to cancer.

My parents were out of town the weekend of the party, which actually worked out well since we wanted to keep it small—if they were around we would have had to invite half of Huntington. We still had it at their house, though, so it was like we were back in high school, only now instead of stealing the alcohol from them, we bought it using their credit card—one of the many benefits of getting older (and having cancer). Melissa's best friend, Sherry, and I made a ton of hors d'oeuvres, Ysrael set up the bar, Nick took care of the music and all of Melissa's friends showed up ready to drink to her health.

Halfway through the night, Melissa called everyone into the living room and gave a little speech. She thanked all of her friends for coming to the party and for being there for her over the past six months. "I love you guys," she said as she raised her glass. Then, as she began to give a special thank you to Ysrael and Andrew—who was asleep upstairs—she started crying. "I am so lucky to have the best husband and the best baby in the world," she said, trying to catch her breath. "I just can't imagine having to do this without them." It was the only time I had seen Melissa cry since she'd been diagnosed and it made me—and everyone else in the room—cry too. As Ysrael hugged her, Melissa wiped away her tears and said, "OK, let's keep drinking!"

Melissa's end-of-treatment party happened to fall on the second anniversary of my diagnosis, a coincidence I mentioned only to Nick so as not to take away from Melissa's special night. Still, I obsessed about it. It was so weird to think that she was diagnosed more than a year after me and she was already seemingly through with cancer. I had had CML for two years and I was still popping my pills, still not knowing what the hell was going to happen to me. She and I used to talk about who had it worse and on that night, I really believed that I did. Sure, she had to go through chemo and radiation, but it was all over now. Her hair was growing back and she was even talking about when she and Ysrael were going to have their next child—September 2005 was the plan (she wasn't worried at all about the effects of the nitrogen mustard; she could "feel" that she was still fertile). For me, having children was still a giant question mark, and there was a good chance I would never be able to put my cancer behind me.

I really shouldn't have been complaining. I was feeling great, my leukemia was still undetectable (which meant I was in remission, even if it was qualified by the fact that I was still being treated) and I had five million of my own "healthy" stem cells on ice. After my last biopsy came back showing that my cancer was all but gone, Dr. Mauro had suggested harvesting my stem cells and freezing them for a rainy day. It was doubtful that I'd ever use them—if I relapsed, I would get Meghan's stem cells, not my own—but it was a good thing to have them anyway. If my body rejected Meghan's stem cells, I could be given back my own to at least reset the clock. Or there could be some experimental treatment developed someday using patients' own stem cells. Either way it couldn't hurt, so my mom and I headed back out to OHSU for the procedure.

The whole thing was done on an outpatient basis. After a few days of giving myself injections of a drug to boost my cell count, my mom and I (and John, the photographer) went to the hospital. Nurses put an "out" line in my left hand and an "in" line in my right arm and hooked me up to a giant whirring machine. For three hours I had to lie there completely still while my blood got taken out, run through the machine so that the stem cells could be separated and collected, and then put back in. I had to squeeze a little squishy globe the whole time so that my vein wouldn't collapse. John thought this was very funny and spent most of the time singing "She's got the whole world in her hand." I tried to laugh with him, but I wasn't amused. My veins burned and my arms were so stiff from holding them straight that I thought I might puke. And the machine kept beeping and vibrating and, if I stopped squeezing the world, making a horrible flatlining-like sound.

Getting the required 5 million stem cells could have taken up to five days on that machine, but I was able to do it in one, thank God. I was just so physically and emotionally drained that

I couldn't have handled another day. Especially after what went down once I left the hospital. First, I had to stop at Rite Aid to get a few different medications to counter the side effects from the harvest (low calcium and low platelet counts). There was no parking outside so my mom hovered while I ran in, still wobbly from the procedure. After I waited in line for 20 minutes, the pharmacist told me he couldn't get me any of the medications I needed. Jerk. Then, on my way out, some kid about my age with designer clothes and tattoos all over his face asked me for money, then cursed at me when I said "sorry" and walked by. I wanted to turn around and say, "I have cancer you waste of life, you should be giving *me* money." Instead I just put on my sunglasses and cried.

When we finally got back to the hotel—which took a while since my mom got caught in a series of one-way streets that sent us over a bridge and onto the freeway—I was really frustrated. My mom dropped me off so I could go up to the room while she parked the car, but when I got into the elevator and pressed the button for our floor, it didn't light up. I pressed it again and again but it just wasn't working. By this point I was really upset—and fortunately alone—so I just made a fist and punched my knuckle into the button as hard as I could a few times. The elevator moved, but my knuckle started gushing blood. By the time I got to my room, my finger had blown up to twice its normal size.

When my mom came into the room and saw me lying on the bed crying, finger bleeding, she told me I should see a therapist. I told her I'd put it on my to-do list. She was probably right, though. Every time I had to do any cancer activity that was more complicated than popping my pills, I'd find an excuse to freak out—my jeans were too tight, the room-service brownie wasn't homemade like they said it would be, Nick refused to take a walk with me—and punch a wall or throw something. It was a definite pattern. Perhaps having cancer really was getting to me. Maybe these were the side effects. I got to keep my hair, but lose my mind.

A few weeks before Christmas, we were all down in Tennessee for Meghan's graduation. She had actually finished college and she was only a semester behind the rest of her class. Her degree was in American Studies, which none of us—including Meghan—had any clue how to translate into the real world, but we were all thrilled for her. After enduring a three-hour-long ceremony, we celebrated with a big, boozy dinner party back at her apartment (which, for the record, was bigger and nicer than any place Melissa and I had ever lived). A bunch of her friends came over and my dad cooked pork tenderloin, mashed potatoes and Caesar salad. The fire was roaring (she had a fireplace!) and the food was delicious, but the highlight of the evening was meeting the new guy Meghan was dating.

He was the first guy Meghan had gone out with since Dustin and she said she really liked him, so we all tried to too. Melissa clicked with him immediately, which seemed odd. Usually, she's a tough critic. She didn't even like Nick when she first met him—she said he whined too much—and everyone loves Nick. (The "whining" turned out to be just his Midwestern accent.) It wasn't until I overheard Melissa and the boyfriend talking that I realized why they clicked. Melissa was telling him the epic fairy tale of how she and Ysrael had met and fallen in love—and he was listening. For Melissa, interest in her was all it took. I wasn't quite as easy to win over. I tried to make friendly conversation with him throughout the night, but he didn't laugh at my jokes and he answered all my questions with one-word shrugs. I thought he was kind of a jerk. And I was right.

Later that night, Meghan pulled me into the bathroom to tell me about a conversation she and the new boyfriend had just had. Apparently, he told Meghan that he was concerned about getting into a serious relationship with her because of her family's "history" with cancer. Ouch. I had never thought of our diseases that way and it had never occurred to me that our family was now tainted. As I watched the tears well up her eyes, I wanted to go kill the bastard. It was one thing if our cancer limited our lives, but I didn't want it to limit Meghan's, especially when she was just starting a new chapter. But at the same time, I kind of understood where he was coming from. I certainly wouldn't want to date a person who had two sisters with cancer—how depressing. Still, I was totally insulted. Meghan was funny and beautiful and smart (she had really grown up in that last year), and we were the best family ever. Any guy would be lucky to be a part of it. So what if we had cancer, we were still fun, we were still crazy, we were still drinking wine for crying out loud!

When I told Nick, who already didn't like the guy, he wanted to kick his ass. So did Melissa. Instead, we just dodged him for the rest of the night. This got considerably easier after around 11 p.m. when the dude passed out drunk on the couch in the middle of the party. That pretty much sealed the deal. Melissa and I agreed that we'd be picking out Meghan's boyfriends from then on. It was so strange to think that someone of my own flesh and blood, someone who had the same freakin' marrow as me, could have such bad taste in men, but she did.

Breaking up with the loser guy, which Meghan promptly took care of the next morning, didn't cause her too much pain. She was leaving Tennessee for good and coming back to New York to be Andrew's nanny. This wasn't her life goal, of course, but she wanted to help Melissa, who'd be starting to work full time again in January. We were all excited to have Meghan back home and grateful to her for what she was doing. As it turned out, she'd be making almost as much as I was making at *Glamour*, so it wasn't that much of a sacrifice. Plus, she'd get to spend every day with Andrew, and nothing could be better than that.

Christmas was the usual chaos, but it was extra special chaos because Nick was finally with us. Having him around to open presents and complain about going to church and get yelled at by my dad for not opening the flue made the holiday—and our family—seem complete. Melissa kept joking that maybe my Christmas present from him would be an engagement ring, but I knew we weren't in danger of that happening. The thought had occurred to Nick, but not in a serious way. "Do you think they're all hoping I'll put on my Santa hat and my matching pajamas and get on one knee under the tree and propose to you while the dogs hump my leg?" he asked with a grin. "They'd love it," I said, laughing. We both knew we'd rather die than have my family watch us get engaged, but we also knew that we wanted to do it. It was no longer a taboo subject for us. Suddenly, everything just felt right.

The marriage talk was precipitated by the fact that Nick had finally gotten a new job. This was a huge milestone for us, but it didn't happen quite the way we had planned. After getting up the courage to tell my dad that he needed to leave the company, and Huntington, Nick started looking for a new job. My dad seemed OK with this at first, but after about two months of Nick's job searching, he freaked. It was a Sunday night and we were all my parents' house for dinner. Nick told my dad that he had an interview the next day so he'd be coming in late. My dad asked him who the interview was with and, jokingly, Nick said it was with one of my dad's biggest competitors. Big mistake. My dad flipped. He told him—screamed at him, actually—that this was *not* the way it worked in the real world, and that he couldn't keep missing work to go on job interviews and that he had two weeks to clean out his desk. He was fired. Fired! Right there in the kitchen while Melissa was setting the table and my mom and

I were making a pear and goat cheese salad. We were all stunned.

My dad stormed upstairs and Nick just sat there for a second looking like he'd seen a ghost. "Holy shit," was all the rest of us could say. "Well, I guess I'm going to go back to my apartment," Nick said, laughing nervously. My mom told him he should just stay for dinner, that my dad wouldn't be back down, but I knew he wanted out of there—and rightfully so. I told him that I'd stay and finish making dinner (I was in the middle of dredging chicken at that point) and bring our plates over to his place in a little while. My mom, who was equally devastated by my father's behavior, insisted on coming with me to make sure Nick knew how much she and my dad loved him and to remind him that my dad just gets crazy sometimes.

As with most of my father's tantrums, we knew his flip out on Nick came from a good place. My dad didn't want to lose him. He had invested time and money and caring into Nick and I think he truly believed that he was going to stay with him forever, that we'd all live happily ever after in Huntington. If it were up to him, he would build three little houses in the backyard for each of his daughters' families to live in and we'd all meet at his house every night for dinner. "*We'll* do that," Melissa would say whenever my dad brought up his fantasy plan. Nick and I, however, wouldn't. We loved my family but we needed some separation, we needed our own life.

So, after my father apologized for firing Nick in the kitchen, they came up with an arrangement that suited both of them. Nick would start his own little company in Manhattan, doing the same thing he was doing for my father's company—selling through them and using all of the same resources—but he wouldn't have a salary or a boss. He'd make his own hours and work on straight commission, like an independent contractor. A few years back this would have made me nervous—no paycheck unless he works his ass off—but I knew he could do it.

He found office space in Manhattan and signed a lease to start on the first of the year. It was the perfect plan.

A few days after Christmas, my mom, Meghan, Melissa, Andrew and I headed down to Miami for a quick getaway. The trip was Melissa's and my idea as a way to say goodbye to a crazy year and celebrate all the good things that had happened for us. Melissa was in remission, I was in molecular remission, Meghan had graduated from college and my mom had kept it all together. She was the one who really deserved the vacation.

I knew that having a sick child was my mom's worst nightmare, so having two must have been a living hell for her. But she managed to stay calm and positive for the rest of us. And she never lost her sense of humor. "I'm going to have to be committed to the nuthouse after this is all over," she'd say, smiling and shaking her head at the same time. "It's like I'm living one of my bad novels. Maybe *I* should write a book!" Most importantly, she stayed by our sides. She gave up whatever she was doing to come to our appointments with us and pick up our prescriptions for us and call our insurance companies to argue over bills. Her life revolved almost completely around her daughters' cancer and she never complained. She would do anything in the world for us if it meant we'd get well again.

Originally, Ysrael was going to watch Andrew, so it could be just the girls, but then Melissa and my mom decided that he had to come with us. It wasn't that they didn't trust Ysrael to take care of him, it was just that they didn't want to leave him alone with the baby for three whole days and nights (in other words, they didn't trust Ysrael to take care of him). We were only there for a few days, but it was totally worth it. We lay at the beach from 10 a.m. to 6 p.m. every day and drank mojitos and ate yummy food. I was doing an "ab challenge" for the magazine—a six week workout plan that was supposed to give me a six-pack—so I had to work out every day and limit myself to one banana daiquiri on the beach (or risk looking fat in my "after" photo) but that was OK. I was just happy to be surrounded by the three women I loved most. I felt lucky just to be there. Melissa did too. And even though we didn't know what the future would bring for either of us, for those few days, we were happy and healthy and hopeful.

11 The end (sort of)

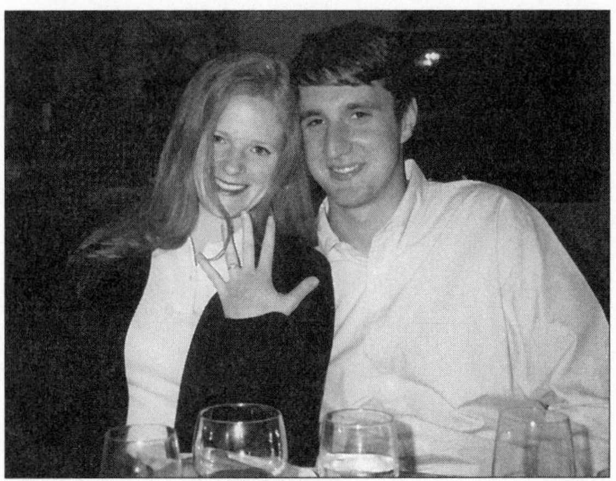

Nick and me the night after we got engaged

On a Wednesday morning in the beginning of March, my phone rang a little too early for it to be Melissa calling to recap who got fired on *The Apprentice*. My heart dropped as I reached for the receiver. Even though I'd had that feeling a million times before, I just knew something was up. I was right. "Grandma Ruth died this morning," my mom said. "When? How? Is Daddy OK?" I asked as I started sobbing into the phone. Grandma Ruth was 83 and she had told me herself only weeks earlier that she was ready to go, but still, I couldn't believe she was gone. And I hated that I didn't get to say goodbye.

I cried more in the days after that phone call than I ever had in my life. Other than my Uncle Bud, who died of a sudden heart attack when I was a freshman in college, I had never lost anyone close to me. And this was my Grammy. My father was beyond sad, too. For whatever pain she may have caused him in his life, he and his mom were really close. He was constantly calling her and running over to see her just to check in. And even though he may have acted like his daily visits were a chore sometimes, I knew he was really going to miss them. "It just feels so strange to think that I won't be seeing her today," he said the next morning when I got to the house. "I can't believe I don't have any parents left." I couldn't even look at him without choking up.

Fortunately, my family knew all too well how to make the most of a sad situation. We all pulled together and had a great send-off weekend for Grandma Ruth. Since I was the both the writer and the speaker in the family, my father and my aunts asked me to give the eulogy. Grandma Ruth wasn't always the best mother but she was an awesome grandmother so it made sense coming from the grandkids' perspective. I was a little reluctant at first (such a big responsibility, so nerve-wracking—couldn't I just be allowed to be sad?), but I knew I had to do it for Grammy. I loved her so much and even though she had been getting older and sicker over the past few years and I didn't get to see her a lot, we were still really close. She still read everything I wrote and gave me recipes and book recommendations and great advice. She still called me her gem.

I knew that the eulogy was the most important speech I'd ever give and it had to be perfect. And it was. Even my delivery was flawless. The only time I almost lost it was when I talked about Mrs. Peach. That was my grandma's screen name when we used to host make-believe cooking shows. Before she moved to New York full time, she used to come up from Florida just for the summers and stay with my family. She was a really good cook and soups—cream of celery, beef barley, split pea—were her specialty. Every time she'd make one, she and I would pretend we were on TV. She was the host, Mrs. Peach, and I was her lovely assistant Charlotte. We'd take out all of the ingredients and line them up on the counter in a very precise way and then she'd say, "Charlotte—what's the first rule of cooking?" And I'd answer dutifully, "Wash your hands and always start with a clean surface!" We'd even take commercial breaks and do the *Frugal Gourmet* smell test where you waft the aroma toward you using your hand instead of sticking your face in the pot (which wasn't allowed in Mrs. Peach's kitchen). We hadn't hosted a cooking show in years but we reminisced about it a lot. And I would really miss that.

Somehow in the days after her death I felt closer to my grandma than I'd felt in years. And as I talked to all of my cousins and my sisters about what they'd remember and miss most about Grammy, I realized something about her—and me. My Grandma had a real joie de vivre. She traveled the world—she'd been everywhere from Bangladesh to Budapest—and ate decadent foods and always saved room for dessert (cheesecake and tiramisu were her favorites) and bought expensive and beautiful things for herself and everyone she loved. Even though her husband had died in a plane crash when she was just 52 years old, she lived the rest of her life to its absolute fullest. She did what made her happy and she didn't care what anyone said about that.

And I knew then that I had to do the same. I had a renewed sense of life after the funeral. Sometimes it was easy for me to forget that I still had a pretty big question mark on my timeline, that I could relapse tomorrow and need a transplant, that I could die. I thought I knew what all of those "life is short" and "life is precious" clichés meant, but after losing my grandma it really hit me. Even though I never *felt* sick from the CML, I had been sick and the Gleevec had given me a second chance at life. And I had to make that life one that I was proud of. I had to make every day count. I'm not saying I was going to stop forcing myself to hit the treadmill every morning or watching *The Bachelor* or trying to be a success. But I wouldn't worry so much about pleasing other people. I would take the time to relax, to smell (and taste) the cheeseburgers, to think about what I really wanted. For me. One thing I knew that I wanted was to spend less time with my to-do list and more time with the people I loved. I also knew, now more than ever, that I would love Nick for life, that I wanted to spend the rest of my life with him.

And he felt the same way about me. About a month later, Nick asked me to marry him. It was so exciting and so wonderful and so perfect—not fairytale movie perfect, but perfect for us. My roommate was away so Nick was spending the week at my apartment (his new office was only a few blocks away). I had gotten home from work late that night and neither of us felt like cooking, so Nick suggested we try this little Italian place in my neighborhood that we had always thought looked good. It was a bit fancy for a Tuesday night, but I figured so what? You only live once. And pancetta-wrapped monkfish is even better than a cheeseburger.

We had a great dinner, and just as our tiramisu arrived, Nick got all cute and self-conscious and asked, "Do you really want to marry me?" When he'd asked that question before, I'd just say, "Yeah, don't you want to marry me?" but this time I launched into a million reasons why we should be together forever. Maybe it was the wine, but for some reason I kept going on and on. I told him that he was the best friend I'd ever had and that we'd been through more in our relationship than most married couples go through in a lifetime and we always managed to not only keep it together but to learn from it and love each other more somehow. "We're both better people when we're together," I said, "and I can't imagine not being with you forever."

Nick just sat there and listened, nodding and smiling at everything I said. "Plus, we're really in too deep to turn back now so we might as well just do it," I added, to avoid sounding like a big sap. "Even though we've been together almost five years, I still get excited when an e-mail from you pops up in my inbox at work," I went on. And I guess that clinched it, because he stopped me and said, "I can't believe I'm going to do this right here." My body went numb. He told me he had something for me and pulled a little box out of his pocket. (He had just made *me* give the proposal speech!) The rest is a bit fuzzy, but apparently he asked me to marry him and I said yes.

It's hard to say I was completely surprised. We had gone ring shopping the week before and I showed him the exact one I wanted—a gorgeous antique (that I'd been eyeing for months). I was just surprised that he had done it so soon. And in a packed restaurant! I didn't even know he had that kind of money. I should never have underestimated him. He was working hard and his business was going really well.

As he put the ring on my finger we were both shaking and giggling and trying desperately not to make a huge scene. We quickly paid our check and spent the rest of the night walking around the city hugging and kissing and marveling at our new state. "Holy shit, we're engaged! We're freakin' engaged!" we kept saying. I couldn't take my eye off the ring and when we ducked into a bar for champagne (which the bartender gave us on the house) I told him that I felt bad because I got this awesome diamond and he gets nothing. "Don't feel bad for me," he said. "I get you." After about an hour of enjoying our little secret, we called my family. They knew about Nick's plan—he had asked both my parents for their blessing over the weekend—and they'd been waiting eagerly by the phone. Good news was a very hot commodity at the Zammetts'.

"You know what this means, right?" I said when we got into bed that night.

"Yup," he said, giving me a look and laughing.

"I can die now!" I said.

It sounds morbid, but Nick and I used to talk about how if I died before we got engaged, he'd just be the sad boyfriend. He was so much more than that, of course, but as the boyfriend he wouldn't get the sympathy he deserved. He probably wouldn't even make the obituary. Thirty years down the road when he'd tell people that his old girlfriend died of leukemia, they'd think, "Well, she was only a girlfriend, get over it!" But now I was his fiancée. And since I wasn't planning on dying any time soon, I'd also be his wife. And that was pretty cool. It really seemed like we had our happy ending. It was like a "we showed you" to the cancer gods. Sure, I have this disease, but I can still be in love and get married and live happily ever after.

Of course, happily ever after doesn't always last very long in the real world. A few weeks after our engagement, Nick and I went with Melissa, Ysrael and Andrew to Melissa's friend Sherry's condo on the east end of Long Island. The boys played golf and the girls (and little boy) went wine tasting, one of Melissa and Sherry's favorite weekend activities. Melissa had a nagging cough and as the day went on it seemed to get worse and worse. "My cancer is probably back," she said as she swilled a glass of pinot noir at the fourth winery. If this were the old Melissa, we'd chalk off this statement to her hypochondria, but now that she really did have something to worry about, we couldn't just roll our eyes and ignore her.

"Call your doctor," Sherry and I urged in unison as we put down our wine glasses and stared, open-mouthed, at Melissa. Melissa just wrinkled her nose at the wine (she was more of a white-wine girl) and said she wasn't going to worry about it because she had just gotten a clean bill of health in January. "Plus," she said, "if my cancer's back, I don't want to know about it." Melissa and Ysrael had just closed on a house after months and months of searching. And they were about to pick up their new golden retriever puppy. Melissa's perfect life was finally getting back on track. Her hair had even grown back enough for her to be able to pull it into a tiny ponytail.

Later that night, while Sherry and I were alone, we talked about how concerned we were. Even though I was the one who was still being treated and I was the one who had the far less curable kind of cancer, I always worried more about Melissa. Probably because I believed that if only one of us could be cured, it should be her. When I watched her with Andrew, I just couldn't imagine her not being there to see him grow up. She loved him so much and he loved her so much and the thought of anything happening to her was just too awful to fathom.

About a week later, Melissa called her nurse to get a letter that she needed for her insurance company. Before they hung up, the nurse asked Melissa how she was feeling and Melissa told her about the cough. The next day, she was at the hospital for a chest X-ray—just to be on the safe side, the nurse said. We all tried to stay calm as we waited for her to call with the results, but it wasn't easy. What if her cancer's back? I couldn't help thinking every five minutes. I had always had a feeling it would come back but I never thought it would happen this soon. I suddenly felt really guilty for ever saying I was envious of her remission, or of her quicker treatment. I should have known better. In some ways, achieving remission is the hardest part of having cancer. At least during treatment, while you're feeling sick and tired and being poked and prodded, you know you're doing something to fight it. When that's over, all you can do is wait and wonder and obsess about what the next test result will bring.

"I'm fine!" Melissa said when she called me a few minutes after the X-ray. Fortunately, the doctor had read it immediately and it was clean. Unfortunately, that wasn't the end of it. A few days later, the doctor called Melissa to say that the radiologist had taken a closer look at the X-ray and had seen a spot near Melissa's heart. They needed her to come back right away and have a CAT scan.

By the time Melissa got to the hospital for the test, we

were all convinced she had relapsed—how can you not think the worst when the worst has already happened twice?

Melissa was sure of it too. She called me in tears as she left the test wondering how she'd be able to pay her mortgage if she had to go through chemo again and couldn't work. "I'll lend you money, Melis," I said, then added, "but I really don't think your cancer is back." She didn't believe me and after trying to convince her for a few more minutes, I finally just conceded. "You know what? If you have cancer again, you'll treat it again and beat it again."

But it didn't come to that. A few days later Melissa found out that the spot was just scar tissue. No more cancer for Melissa. At least for now.

On May 20th, 2004, Andrew turned one year old. He had a *Finding Nemo*-themed birthday party with a Nemo ice cream cake and Nemo goody bags for all his friends. Nick and I bought him one of those Little Tikes play castles, complete with flag, tower and slide. I'm his godmother and I knew that the main reason Melissa picked me over Meghan was because I'd always have a job and be able to give him the best presents (the real role of a godparent according to her). It was his first birthday and I had to come through. Fortunately, Nick was making good money so he sprang for the $300 gift. I bought the card. I had been promoted to associate editor at *Glamour* but I wasn't exactly rolling in the dough yet.

Meghan was still nannying for Andrew, but she wouldn't be for much longer. She loved hanging out with him and being there to see him crawl for the first time and walk for the first time and point to his ear when you asked him where his nose was (I was completely jealous). But she was also itching for a new job, one where she was required to get dressed in the morning and actually leave the house. She missed that. She had turned into a diaper-changing, *Baby Einstein*-watching, mashed-carrot feeding mommy. And she was only 21. It didn't help that the new dog Melissa and Ysrael had gotten (and named Hamburg after Hamburg, Germany, the place they consummated their love—gag me) now came as a package deal with Andrew. Melissa would drop them both off at my parents' house (where Meghan was living) each morning and Meghan was expected to not only take care of Andrew but his little dog too. Hamburg was a puppy (and a bad one at that) so Meghan couldn't take her eyes off him. She was constantly taking Andrew's toys—and sometimes Andrew's hands—out of the dog's mouth, chasing after him when he stole her food and, most importantly, making sure she had all his pee cleaned off the dining room floor before my father came home for lunch. It was out of control to say the least.

Fortunately, Meghan had a great outlet. After coming with me for one of my speeches at a kick-off event for Team In Training, the endurance-training arm of the Leukemia & Lymphoma Society, Meghan decided she had to get involved. She would do the San Diego marathon—she'd walk the 26.2 miles (she still had the bum knee from skiing so she never really ran), her friend Tracy would run them, and together they'd raise the necessary funds to participate. I was truly impressed. Just a year earlier the only exercise Meghan got was changing her outfit six times before heading to the bars. She had come a long way from her days of Marlboro Lights and Coors Lights and bad boyfriends.

She'd come so far that I asked her to be my maid of honor. Melissa agreed that it had to be Meghan—it was just too perfect. Not only was she my bone marrow match, but she had also been with Nick and me on our first date (a 311 concert at a bar on the UT campus). She'd known Nick as long as I had and she loved him like a brother from day one. I knew it would be extra special for her. And for me, too. Plus, Melissa was my self-appointed wedding planner, so she'd be running the show anyway and could "pick up any of Meghan's slack." But I didn't think she'd need to. I had a lot of faith in Meghan. By the time she completed the marathon in June, which Nick and I were there to see, Meghan and Tracy had raised more than $15,000 for the Society in honor of Melissa and me. She was a good kid after all.

The rest of the summer was glorious. A few weeks after the marathon, Melissa and Ysrael moved into their new house. My father had spent a month completely gutting and renovating the thing so it was an especially triumphant milestone. And Melissa had worked so hard knocking down and rebuilding walls alongside my dad and Ysrael that she had lost a ton of weight. She was thrilled and couldn't wait to put on a bathing suit and drink margaritas by the pool. "Melissa lives in a fantasy world," my mom would say to me at least once a week. "She doesn't have paint on her walls and she thinks she's going to spend the weekend at Sherry's condo while your father's up at her house busting his ass for her." Fortunately, my dad did take the occasional break. When he'd had enough spackling or wiring for the day (he rarely went to his own office anymore), we'd all go out on the boat and fish and float and relax.

The best part of the summer was that Nick and I set a date for our wedding. This was no easy feat. I was convinced that people must plan their weddings before they're even engaged because trying to find a place for the reception that had the same availability as my church was nearly impossible. And we were looking at dates over a year away! I had never been one of those girls who dreamt about my wedding day—I always fantasized about *being* married, about throwing dinner parties and reading in bed together and taking the kids on vacations, but never about which color linens would be on the tables at the cocktail hour—but suddenly I was really into it. I had no choice. There were so many decisions to be made and since decisions had never been my strong suit, I became obsessed. Fortunately, Melissa was around to tell me what I liked and disliked, which, in the end, worked out perfectly. Nick and I would be getting married in July 2005 at St. Patrick's church in Huntington. The reception would be at a beautiful old mansion on a golf course, where my father was already planning to have a putting contest after we cut the cake. All that was left to do was find my dress—and that was going to be easy.

As luck would have it, Dr. Mauro's wife, Anne, is a bridal gown designer. For years she worked for Yumi Katsura, a high-end bridal company in New York City and she had recently opened a shop of her own in Portland. Dr. Mauro had always joked that someday maybe she'd design my wedding dress, and now someday was here. Her dresses were beautiful and I planned to meet with her about designing one just for me the next time I was in Oregon for a biopsy. Nothing like a little one-stop shopping.

Right before Labor Day, Nick and I moved into an apartment together in the city. I had debated whether I wanted to do the whole living-in-sin thing, but figured what the hell. We'd be married soon anyway. Nick moved his business (which consisted of a desk, a computer and a phone) into the apartment and we started setting up our life together. We couldn't wait to pick out our dishes and our towels and buy our first pumpkin and our first Christmas tree. We were giddy about the future. We should have known better.

A few weeks into September, Melissa and Meghan went to see Melissa's Long Island doctor. She'd had some routine tests done about a week earlier and the results were in. But Melissa wasn't concerned about those. She really just wanted to find out exactly when she could start trying to have another baby. She was feeling great and was wondering if she should start taking folic acid and thinking about going off the Pill soon. Wishful thinking to say the least.

"Melissa relapsed, the cancer is growing fast and she has to have a transplant," Meghan said breathlessly when she called my office from the car on the way back from the appointment. "Whoa, whoa, whoa," I said. "What are you saying?" I had forgotten they were even going to the appointment that day. "You're kidding, right, Meg?" I asked, thinking maybe she was just playing an exceptionally cruel joke. It was just too unbelievable to fathom. But she wasn't kidding. Meghan put Melissa on the phone. "Do you believe this?" Melissa said. "What," I said, pausing, desperately trying not to lose it, "what did they say?" I started sobbing into the phone. I couldn't help it. "What's going to happen? How do they know?" I couldn't catch my breath. Then Melissa started crying. It was September 15, 2004. Not even a year since her remission party and we were back to square one. Again.

The entire pod stared in concern as I wiped my tears and got the details. Apparently, Melissa's PET scan showed a lot of activity in her chest and lungs and abdomen. Her cancer was back and this time it was for real. "And I have Amanda's bachelorette weekend coming up," Melissa said. I had to love that she could think of a party at a time like this. One of Melissa's best friends was getting married soon and Melissa was not only a bridesmaid but also the travel agent extraordinaire for the three-day-long bachelorette party in Orlando. "I planned the whole goddamn thing, Er, I can't miss it."

Melissa's doctor told her that they'd have to biopsy one of her lymph nodes to confirm the diagnosis, but she could pretty much count on lots of chemo and radiation and a stem cell transplant. Soon. Fortunately, with Hodgkin's they mostly do autologous transplants, meaning they use the patient's own stem cells, so Melissa would not need a match—a good thing since we already knew she didn't have one in Meghan or me. It's a grueling procedure, but there was a chance she would be cured forever. "Just a chance Melis? Is that really what she said?" Not surprisingly, the only thing Melissa really retained from the meeting—other than the potential interference with Amanda's bachelorette weekend—was that after the transplant, she definitely wouldn't be able to have any more kids.

"Er, you gotta find me a fertility specialist so I can freeze some embryos," Melissa said to me before I hung up. She didn't have much time and her doctor wasn't even sure it was good idea, but Melissa didn't care. She could take the relapse, but she would not give up her fertility without a fight.

Surviving 12

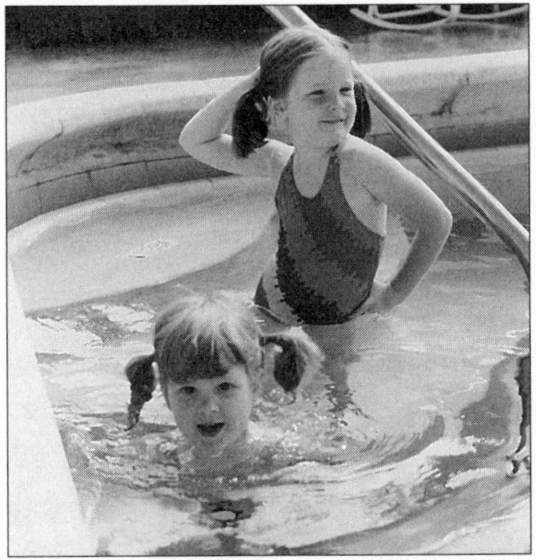

Melissa (striking a pose) and me in the pool at Grandma Ruth's

IT'S HARD NOT TO FEEL BAD FOR YOURSELF, NOT TO finally start asking, "why me?" when cancer hits your family for the third time in three years. We had all gotten pretty good at the shit-happens-we-deal-with-it thing, but very quickly it got much harder to pull off. And to me, Melissa's relapsing was worse than either of us being diagnosed for the first time. When a disease comes back after you thought you had it beat, suddenly there isn't as much hope. Suddenly remission, let alone a cure, seems so much harder to achieve. You've already failed once, what's to say you're not going to fail again?

But another thing happens when cancer comes back. You know what to do and you just do it. You grieve less and act more because that's what you've learned to do. Because there is so much more riding on a relapse. When we found out that

Melissa's cancer was back it was as if everything up to that point was just a dress rehearsal, like we were being called into battle after practicing all this time with rubber bullets on a firing range. I could almost hear the sirens blasting and the commander saying, "This is not a drill." So within minutes of getting the news, we went into action. And that's what kept us sane.

The plan was very clear: Melissa would do a special relapse protocol developed by a special relapse doctor at Sloan-Kettering. To start, she'd have to go into the hospital for three days of heavy-duty chemo. The she'd come out for two weeks to recover. Somewhere during that recovery time she'd have a stem cell harvest, just like the one I'd had, only they wouldn't be sending her stem cells to some remote location; they'd be keeping them close at hand for an eventual transplant. Then more chemo, more recovery and finally a PET scan to see if it had all worked. If she was in remission, they'd go forward with the transplant. If she wasn't, they'd give her two more months of outpatient chemo. But no matter what, she'd be getting the transplant eventually—it's just what they do for Hodgkin's patients who relapse.

"Don't ask me why, but I've been doing some research on transplants," Melissa said a few days after her re-diagnosis. "And for the whole month that I'm in the hospital, I'm not going to be able to see Andrew. Now every time I look at him, I cry." After the extra chemo Melissa would get before the transplant, she'd basically be left with no immune system and that meant no visits from snotty-nosed, drooly babies—even really cute ones like Andrew. But then she'd be given back her own stem cells and she'd grow a new immune system and be OK. It wouldn't be quite that simple. She could count on getting pretty sick and losing her hair all over again and, once she got out of the hospital, being under house arrest for a few months. She'd have to avoid movie theaters, restaurants, shellfish, life.

A transplant was the one big scary thing that had been

haunting me since I'd been diagnosed, and now instead of me, my sister was going to have one. It seemed so unfair, like she was taking the heat for something I had done—which, come to think of it, she never did. Growing up, Melissa was the one who did the bad things—sneaking my dad's car out and driving it to the mall before she even had her permit, drinking 40s of Old English with her friends during her lunch period ("liquid lunch," they called it), cutting school to go to Splish Splash with her crush. I was an angel compared to her. Naturally, the fact that she had done all those things helped me slide by on a few of my own indiscretions, but still, I was by far the most law-abiding of my parents' three girls. I only cut the whole school day once—and I had gotten my mom's permission first. Back then, I was the one who covered for Melissa and I liked being able to protect her. I just wished I could do it now. But so much had changed. Having the boy you like smile at you in the hallway was no longer the most important thing in life. Now we just wanted to make it to 30.

Before Melissa could start the relapse protocol, she had to get an official positive reading on a biopsy. Even though her doctors were sure the cancer was back, they needed to be 110 percent before they discussed the details of her treatment. Not surprisingly, this turned out to be a complete pain in the ass. A few days after her re-diagnosis, Melissa went to Sloan for the biopsy. Her doctors had decided to take it from one of the lymph nodes in her lung, since the procedure to get it from there was the least invasive. The biopsy doctor stuck a tube down Melissa's throat, through her trachea and into her lung. It was called a bronchoscopy and to me it sounded pretty invasive. But Melissa (who said the doctor was so hot she didn't care what he did to her) left with only a sore throat. And the sexy doctor was confident he had gotten what he needed.

He was wrong. A few days later, Melissa went in for her appointment with the fancy relapse specialist, assuming he was ready to talk timeline. Instead, he told her that the bronchoscopy didn't yield any results. The problem was that Melissa had a lot of scar tissue in her lungs left over from her previous radiation. And the spot where she'd relapsed in her abdomen was too small to biopsy. But the doctor had a plan. They'd wait two weeks and hope that the mass in Melissa's abdomen grew big enough to get at with a needle. This sounded nuts to me. Wasn't her cancer moving fast? Didn't we have to do something about it?—but Melissa didn't seem to mind. "Once they get a positive reading it's going to be real, Er," she said. "For now I can just pretend it's not happening." Whatever works.

Part of the reason Melissa had such a good attitude about the whole thing was because she had seven unborn children to celebrate. It sounds unbelievable, like a miracle even, but within two weeks of her diagnosis, she'd been able to put seven healthy embryos on ice. And I'd helped. After I got off the phone with her that first night, all of my podmates came running over to give me hugs and tissues and words of encouragement. Then they went to work on finding Melissa a doctor. Because *Glamour* had done some big investigative stories on women's fertility, our editors had a lot of great contacts in the field. Even better, one of them had a best friend who was a fertility specialist.

Two days later Melissa had an appointment to talk embryos, and it couldn't have worked out more perfectly. After running a bunch of tests, the doctor found out that Melissa's ovaries were still working great. The nitrogen mustard hadn't caused any damage after all. And she was at a point in her menstrual cycle where she could start the hormone injections right away. She did her first shot that night and a week later had her eggs extracted. A few days after that, she had her seven embryos. Nothing could get her down now.

Naturally, no triumph would be complete without its share of setbacks. At first, Ysrael was completely against the idea of freezing embryos. He thought it was creepy and weird and sacrilegious and pointless since they already had one great kid. I actually had to come out to Huntington to administer Melissa's first shot of hormones because Ysrael had refused (and because Melissa wanted a pro). And up until five minutes before they left for the semen-collecting appointment, Melissa had no semen. And no husband. Nick and I had gone to her house the morning of the appointment with egg sandwiches for Melissa and Andrew (we were boycotting Ysrael because he was being such a jerk) and Ysrael was missing. He was gone when Melissa woke up and when she tried to call—about 17 times—he didn't answer his cell phone. Nick and I did our best to keep Melissa calm, but it wasn't easy. "I will absolutely divorce him if he doesn't do this for me," she said. "What's the big fucking deal? All I want is a little sperm. If he's on the golf course, so help me God . . ."

As it turned out, he wasn't playing golf. He was at church trying to find a priest to talk to about his doubts. But because he was still so hard to understand (and by this point it had nothing to do with the language), we were all freaking out. And even though his concerns were valid, we wanted to kill him. Lucky for him, he came around just in time to watch a little porn and race to the appointment. Nick and I stayed with Andrew, heads spinning. "I hope you know I would never do that to you," he said.

"I know," I said, finally taking a bite of my now-cold egg sandwich. "Let's just watch *Blue's Clues*." I needed a break from the drama.

Nick couldn't even talk about Melissa's relapse without getting choked up—and angry. He loved her like she was his own sister and he felt so bad for her, but it was more than that. Knowing that she was going to get sick again and bald again and have a transplant reminded him that someday that could be me. I tried to assure him that I was fine and that I planned to stay that way, but the parallel between my life and Melissa's was just too obvious for any of us to ignore.

Because of the two-week wait-for-the-cancer-to-grow period, Melissa was able to go to Amanda's bachelorette weekend. Of course, since her main doctor had originally told her she'd be starting treatment right away, Melissa had assumed she'd be vomiting and losing weight and had therefore been eating every meal like it was her last. But now three weeks had gone by and she still didn't have a positive biopsy reading, let alone a chemo drip. "I'm so fucking fat!" she said on the phone to me as she packed for Florida. "I can't believe those bastards couldn't give me the chemo before I left. What the hell am I going to wear now?"

I was glad to see the whole perspective thing was stumping her as much as it had stumped me. She was facing a battle for her life—for the second time—and all she could think about was how many sit-ups she'd have to do to get rid of her belly in the next 24 hours. In the end, of course, it didn't matter. Melissa had a blast with her friends. She relaxed by the pool, got a facial, drank wine and laughed at the stripper's saggy thong. It was a great little vacation for her, a calm before her storm. And the best part was that she could play the cancer card whenever she wanted to duck out of the bar early, which she always did. Melissa liked to party, but she also liked to be in bed by 11 p.m. At the latest.

A few days after Melissa got back from Florida, my mom, Meghan and I headed to Portland for my bone marrow biopsy/wedding dress consultation. We felt bad leaving Melissa at home with only the boys, but she was still waiting around for her cancer to grow and I really needed both Meghan and my mom with me (my mom because she's my mom and Meghan because she's my maid of honor and has good taste and I wanted her opinion on my dress). And we were all secretly thrilled to be getting away from the craziness. My mom especially. She had been driving into the city with Melissa for every single appointment and cooking for Melissa and Ysrael every night and constantly babysitting for Hamburg (who was still very bad) and Andrew (who was still very cute but a handful) and my dad, who was not taking the relapse news very well at all.

At first, he was distraught, saying how the whole thing was so awful he couldn't even think about it. But then he got proactive—and holistic. The day after Melissa was diagnosed, he decided that we should all start eating only organic foods. Organic butter, organic bread, organic eggs, organic everything. "Are you going to drink organic martinis?" my mom joked. She believed doctors and medicine were still the best way to heal people, not free-range chicken. My dad did too, he just wanted something to make him feel a little less helpless. So he went to Wild By Nature—a place I could never normally get him into because it was so expensive—and spent $500 on organic chips and cheeses and meats and flax oil and collard greens and dried seaweed. And a few other fun things.

"Daddy is on his way to my house with a wheat grass shot," Melissa said when she called me later that day. "If I'm dying I want to eat Big Macs, not grass."

"You're not dying, Melis," I said. "And it's good for you so just drink it with your Big Mac." Suddenly joking about dying wasn't so funny anymore.

Fortunately for Melissa—and my parents' grocery budget —my dad quickly found a more pressing project and the organic food got phased out. About a week after Melissa's re-diagnosis there was a nasty rainstorm and the flood it caused did major damage to the downstairs bedroom at my parents' house. This was a blessing in disguise to say the least. Within days my father had completely gutted the thing—"It needed to be redone anyway," he said as he pulled up the carpet and ripped down the sheet rock and broke down the closet doors. His plan was to raise the roof, switch two of the windows to maximize the light, put down cement and fancy tiles and rig up an elaborate self-heating system. And it was all he could talk about. He wanted it to be Melissa's "sterile room" when she got out of the hospital from her transplant so it had to be perfect. And considering how much time he spent back there, it would be.

The day we arrived in Portland, Meghan got a call from New York City saying that she'd gotten the job she'd been interviewing for (an ad sales position with a small publishing company in the city). We were all thrilled, no one more than Meghan. She had stopped babysitting for Andrew back in August and had been looking for a job on and off since then. It hadn't been easy, so she was definitely ready for some good news. And ready to finally move out of my parents' house. Though Andrew was at daycare now, Hamburg the terrible still spent the day at my parents'. And with all the construction and the drama over Melissa's diagnosis, it had become an even crazier place to be. Meghan had been planning to move into the city, but without a paycheck, it would have been a little difficult. Now she could do it and she could officially join the real world, business suits and all. And considering we were in no-sales-tax, outlets-galore land, the timing couldn't have been more perfect.

The highlight of our trip was that I was able to make a decision on a wedding dress. We went to see Anne Mauro before we we even went to OHSU and I quickly realized that she was just as kind and gentle as her husband. She was also one of the tiniest people I'd ever met—and she was seven months pregnant at the time. We hung out at her studio for hours, trying on dresses, discussing designs and fabrics and posing for Basil, the new photographer *Glamour* had hired to document the whole thing. By the end of our appointment we had come up with a design that we all loved—a low-cut halter with a band of antique silver beads under the bust.

Anne would make up a formal drawing and send it to me in New York for my approval, and then she'd get started. I'd have to come out to Portland a few months later for my muslin fitting and at least once more for an actual fitting, but I didn't care. I never minded going to Portland and having to go for a fitting was better than having to go for a bone marrow biopsy. Unless of course I didn't lose the ten pounds I was planning to lose before the wedding. In that case I'd probably prefer the biopsy.

My appointment with the other Mauro went well, too. It was so strange to be talking about my cancer again after talking about nothing but Melissa's for so long. I hadn't even thought about my CML in months. Still, I was glad to be getting a check-up and so grateful for Dr. Mauro, who sat and talked to us for two hours, giving us what amounted to a state of the CML address. He started by saying that my counts had been so consistently undetectable over the past year and a half that doing the biopsy was really just a formality. And that up to that point my CML had remained at a level (zero) where I had the lowest possible chance of relapse.

As far as the future went, it looked like I'd be able to stay on Gleevec for a long time. Maybe even a long, long time. And if I couldn't, there were new drugs being developed for patients who build up a resistance to the Gleevec—two were already in trial phase. I'd also always have the transplant to fall back on. Really, I had the best of all possible worlds—for a cancer patient, anyway. There'd always be that uncertainty, that question—"will my cancer come back?"—but I was doing great and I had a great prognosis and Dr. Mauro couldn't be happier with my status.

Then, of course, I asked him about my fertility. I felt bad rocking the remission boat, but now that Nick and I were engaged, I really wanted to talk options, timing, details. Dr. Mauro had done some research for me and said there were definitely some women with CML out there having babies. But to do it, they had to go off the Gleevec to conceive and to carry the baby. Being off the Gleevec for that long was a huge risk and some of them wound up relapsing. They could go right back on the drug once they gave birth, but who knew if it would work again. And for someone like me who was in such a deep remission, and who might conceivably never have a problem with CML again, going off the drug for any reason seemed to him like throwing away a good thing. He said if I weren't doing so well on the Gleevec, he would be more apt to say I should stop and have a baby. But he hated to mess with what we had going. It was another cancer Catch-22. God, how I loved those.

In the end, of course, Dr. Mauro said it would be up to Nick and me. We'd have to weigh the risks and decide if it was worth it. And Dr. Mauro would support and help us with whatever we decided. I already knew Nick wanted nothing to do with risking my life and after watching Melissa relapse and seeing how that was killing was my parents, I knew that I probably wouldn't either. But I really wanted to have babies! Melissa still said she would carry them for me—"I'll just alternate," she said, joking (I think). "One year I'll have one of my embryos and one year I'll have one of yours." Even Meghan said she'd be a surrogate, but I just couldn't help wanting to do it the old-fashioned way. And considering the wedding was still nine months away and I was only 26, we had plenty of time to discuss it. So, the whole fertility thing went back on the back burner—where I kind of liked it.

After the bone marrow biopsy, which was business as usual—except to Meghan who got to meet Mark and his harmonica for the first time— Dr. Mauro told us about a new CML test they were going to run on my blood. It was called the Nested PCR test and it was able to see the leukemia better than anything they'd used before. But, Dr. Mauro warned, because this test was more sensitive, there was a chance my disease could be detectable now. If that were the case, he added, I shouldn't necessarily assume that the cancer was coming back. It could just be that it was always there and the less sensitive tests couldn't see it. All we'd do is continue to watch my counts as we had been.

We wouldn't have the new results for a few weeks, but I wasn't worried. I had come to take all my cancer stuff with a grain of salt. It's easy to do that when your sister is much worse off than you. I had also already decided that if my counts went up by so much as a percentage point, I wasn't going to tell anybody but Nick. I just couldn't bear to give my parents any cancer news that wasn't really good. They were all but crumbling at this point and I didn't want them to worry about me one bit. Plus, Nick and I had become a real team. He was the one I leaned on most now and I knew we could handle anything together.

When we got back from Oregon, Melissa's cancer ball really got rolling. The mass in her stomach had grown as predicted, but it ended up being too close to an artery for them to biopsy. So, they decided to give the lung one more chance. This time, they'd get at it through her ribcage, by puncturing her lung with a little needle. They'd only use local anesthesia so Melissa would be awake for the whole thing. If any of us—Melissa especially—had taken a step back during those days and realized that our life had become one big episode of *ER*, we probably would have freaked. But fortunately, we were in the zone so the blood and guts and gravity of the whole thing didn't get to us.

The procedure went well. It took four different tries, meaning four different holes in Melissa's lungs, but the doctor was sure he got what they needed this time. Melissa was able to distract herself from the giant needles going into her body by naming every single one of her embryos. In her mind, four of them were boys and three were girls. And Isabella Ruth was already her favorite.

"I officially have Hodgkin's again!" Melissa said, truly triumphant, when she called me a few days after the biopsy. "And

I should be able to start chemo next week. Isn't that great?" Melissa was so relieved because finally starting treatment meant she'd be done with the first round of chemo and out of the hospital just in time for Amanda's wedding.

My parents weren't quite as thrilled with the news. I think my mom was honestly hoping that the doctors had made a mistake, that when they finally got a good enough biopsy it would come back negative, that they'd say it was scar tissue just like they'd said the last time—then again, the last time they may have been wrong about that. My father was happy to have some answers, to finally know what we were dealing with, but that also made him sad. "Now it's real," he said. A few days later he decided to rip up the back deck and redo it with mahogany planks.

Melissa's first round of chemo was pretty rough on her. In addition to having the drugs, she had to have surgery to put a port in a vein right below her neck. When Melissa first found out about this, she flipped—not because she was afraid of the operation, but because she was afraid the tubes that came out of the contraption would show when she wore her bridesmaid's dress for Amanda's wedding the following weekend. But she had to have it. She'd be able to get her future chemo treatment through there and have her stem cell harvest through there and though it seemed—and looked—like something out of Frankenstein, it would actually make her life with cancer a lot easier. By the evening she had warmed to the idea but asked the nurse if she could wait until the next morning to get the surgery. She didn't want to miss *Survivor*.

"I'm starting to feel really sorry for myself," she said to me when I went up to Sloan to visit her the day after her surgery. Her port left her in pain, the medication she was taking to counter the pain made her nauseated, the anti-nausea pills made her really drowsy and the chemo did all three. "This sucks," she said as she turned off *Oprah* and closed her eyes. I didn't know what to say to her because it really did suck. How can you put a positive spin on something that was so obviously negative? Instead of trying, I just told her how Meghan, who had slept over the night before, got on the wrong subway to work that morning and didn't realize it until she was all the way on the Upper West Side. We laughed, then she rolled over and I left. I glanced at the potato chips I'd brought her (sour cream and onion Ruffles just like she'd asked)—they were still sitting unopened on the windowsill—and I started to cry. I couldn't help it. I missed my sister.

But Melissa was a trouper. Though she spent the whole week after her chemo lying in her bed, she made it to Amanda's wedding. And the shawl of her dress covered the port perfectly. She looked beautiful (and, as she pointed out, 11.5 pounds thinner) and even danced the salsa with Ysrael. It was only for a minute—and she later told me it was just so I'd have something positive to write about in my *Glamour* column—but it was great to see. And my whole family was there to watch. Well, everyone except my dad who was on a long-planned golf outing with friends down in Florida. He was bummed he'd be missing the wedding—especially since the rest of us were going—but I think it was a good thing he wasn't there. It was an emotional night and though he was getting better, emotions still weren't his strong suit.

The wedding was held at a beautiful hotel and about an hour before the reception ended, Melissa snuck out and went up to her room. She was exhausted and she didn't want to push herself any more than she already had. She needed to go to bed. Then, not even three minutes after she left, the band came on and said that the bride and groom wanted to dedicate a special song: "Melissa and Ysrael, please join Amanda and Josh on the dance floor," the guitarist said and then launched into Melissa and Ysrael's wedding song—"Hero" by Enrique Iglesias. I went running up to Amanda before she could get on the dance floor to tell her that Melissa had gone upstairs. She just shrugged and said, "OK, so you just dance with Ysrael." (She was a surprisingly calm bride.) So I grabbed Ysrael, who already had tears in his eyes, and we danced cheek to cheek. Meanwhile, Sherry ran to the nearest phone and called up to Melissa's room. Then she told the band to drag out the song for as long as they could. Melissa wouldn't want to miss a dance with her husband—cancer or no cancer.

The rest of the party joined us on the dance floor—Nick asked my mom to dance—and a few minutes later, just as the band was singing, "let me kiss away the pain" and "I will stand by you forever" for the hundredth time, Melissa came running through the ballroom door. Her dress was half unbuttoned in the back but she had made it. I quickly stepped aside and just tried not to cry too much. Melissa and Ysrael only got to dance for about a minute, but it was totally worth it. Seeing them with their arms wrapped around each other, whispering the lyrics into each other's ears, I just knew Melissa was going to be OK.

Later that week Dr. Mauro called to say that my leukemia was undetectable on all tests—including the new Nested test. I couldn't be in better shape. Of course this was cancer news I did want to share with my family and for the first time in a long time, we all felt like celebrating. Because of the massive renovation going on at my parents' house, there was a moratorium on home-cooked Sunday night dinners, so instead we went out to a fancy restaurant in Huntington.

"Here's to staying below the radar," my dad said when we had all gotten our wine glasses filled. He also toasted to Melissa getting well again and Meghan's new job and the new back room, "which is going to be the neatest thing you've ever seen," but all I really remember now is how crazy it was to be sitting there, healthy. I had just passed the three-year anniversary of my diagnosis and I couldn't believe so much time had gone by. I also couldn't believe that after all we'd been through we were right back to where we started. But as I looked around the table, I realized that we really weren't. Melissa had a family and a house (and a dog) and Nick and I had a big wedding to plan and Meghan had a great job (and a new guy she liked who was totally not weird). Our family had grown closer and stronger and we had proven to ourselves, not once, not twice, but three times over that we could face anything life threw our way. And as we clinked glasses and opened our menus, I knew we could—and would—survive. We had to.

Acknowledgments

WHEN I USED TO FANTASIZE ABOUT SOMEDAY WRITING a book, the first thing I would think about writing was the acknowledgments page. I've just always been so lucky to have so many incredible, generous people in my life that I couldn't wait to have a forum to thank them, and to tell them, officially, how grateful I am for their love and support.

That said, there aren't enough pages in this book to mention every person who has touched my life. But here are a few without whom this book would not be possible: My agents, Ed Victor and William Clark; my editor, Tracy Carns, and everyone at The Overlook Press, especially Peter Mayer, Sarah Rosenbloom and David Mulrooney; everyone at *Glamour*, especially Cindi Leive, who gave me the opportunity to share my story and in doing so made my life with cancer better than my life without it, also Jill Herzig, Ellen Seidman, Susan Goodall, Amy Peck, Meg D'Incecco, Cynthia Harris, Catherine Perry, Daryl Chen, Jennifer Peters, Laurie Sandell, Molly Janik Gulati, Alison Ward Frank, Christy Whitney, Amanda Meigher, John Brennan, Dan Hallman and Ronnie Andren; and my friends and colleagues Donald Robertson, Jaimee Zanzinger, Dana Kahn Cooper, Karen Travers, my fairy bookmothers Lindy Hess and Sara Nelson, and Kevin Buckley, who inspires me to do big things simply by believing in me.

There are many people I would never have met had it not been for my diagnosis and I am so thankful that they are in my life: Pia Awal, Kris Carr, Basil Childers, Scott Matz; everyone at the Leukemia & Lymphoma Society, especially Dolores Swirin, Donna Canzano and Stacy Mitz; everyone at The G&P Foundation, especially Denise Rich; everyone at The Marrow Foundation, especially Keri Christensen; everyone at Novartis; all of the nurses at OHSU, especially Mark Browne; all of the *Glamour* readers who wrote letters to me—you are in my thoughts always; and, of course, my doctors Kathleen Cathcart, Brian Druker and especially Michael Mauro. I only wish that every person with cancer could be treated by such a special man. Thank you for everything, Dr. Mauro.

I also want to thank all of the people who have been there for my family over the past few years—whether it's making a phone call or a casserole or a donation, what you do has meant so much to us and we couldn't have survived without your generosity. A special thanks to Donna McNaughton, Rose Melillo, and to the Cittadini family, for giving us a home away from home.

Finally, a very special thanks to the following people:

Alison Brower, the best boss, editor, and mentor a girl could hope for. Thank you for always being there to answer all my questions—and thank you for answering them honestly.

Lauren Smith Brody, an amazing editor, but an even better friend. Your selflessness, dedication and talent blow me away, and without your round-the-clock enthusiasm and encouragement I would never have finished this book. I can only hope that someday I get the opportunity to be as good a friend to you as you've been to me.

Ysrael and Andrew, for loving Melissa as much as I do.

My parents, John and Cindy, for giving me a childhood I love revisiting and the toughness to tackle whatever my adulthood may bring.

And Nick, my best friend. I can't wait to start the next chapter together.

For more information on leukemia, lymphoma and other cancers, or to find out how you can help patients by donating time or money, I recommend the following websites:

The Leukemia & Lymphoma Society
www.leukemia-lymphoma.org

The Marrow Foundation
www.themarrowfoundation.org

The G&P Foundation for Cancer Research
www.gpfoundation.com

Cancer*Care*
www.cancercare.org